Basic Concepts of Track and Trace System for Pharmaceutical Industry

OrangeBooks Publication

Smriti Nagar, Bhilai, Chhattisgarh - 490020

Website: **www.orangebooks.in**

First Edition, 2021

ISBN: 978-93-90837-37-3

Printed in India

BASIC CONCEPTS OF
TRACK AND TRACE
SYSTEM FOR
PHARMACEUTICAL
INDUSTRY

RAMESHWAR VERMA

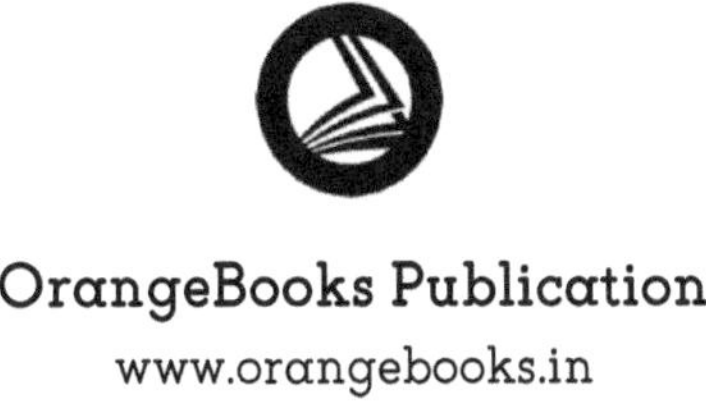

OrangeBooks Publication

www.orangebooks.in

Contents

Chapter | 1

Introduction Of Track And Trace System

Introduction

One of the essential requirements for a drug is the assurance of its quality, together with its efficacy and safety. In the pharmaceutical industry, professionals try to develop and improve analytical methods to assure prescribed treatment will improve patient life quality. On the other side, the patients have to trust in pharmaceutical company's integrity and acknowledge their concern regarding drugs safety. To achieve this ideal, quality of medicine, it is the most challenging mission in the drug development field. A collective joint effort between authorities from all over the world was made to ensure the patient's safety in the 21 century. World Health Organization (WHO), Food and Drug Administration (FDA), European Union (EU) and International Council for Harmonisation of Technical Requirements for Pharmaceuticals for Human Use (ICH) gathered in their guidelines a common purpose. The goal is to help future research projects to find what their background was when they assure the quality of drugs and what can be used for developing new methodological decisions in upgrading the pharmaceutical industry. Every country applies general practices for drug assurance quality based on the submitted regulations. Essentially, there is a national compendium of good manufacturing practices (GMP) with specific chapters and annexes that maintain regulatory obligations.

One of the recent requirements to improve drugs quality is their traceability. Drug serialization is a practice that assures a unique recognition number for every drug unit. The given number may be used for product tracking and authentication in the distribution chain, allowing counterfeits identification. It requires support and collaboration from all partners involved in medicine's marketing. There are several essential elements to be introduced in a serial number: a product code capable of giving essential characteristics like name, pharmaceutical form, concentration, package, batch number, expiration date, and a serial number obtained by a computerized algorithm. This serial number has to be unique and cannot be repeated for at least five years since its introduction on the market.

Technologies have a significant impact in combating counterfeiting drugs process. Nowadays, it is straightforward to manufacture a product which may pass at first glance as an original. Also, the online drugs market (known as a grey market) is very accessible. Accelerated growth of the online pharmacies number could put people's lives in danger. Consequently, serialization process becomes a universal tool as a primary procedure in combatting counterfeiting.

Pharmaceutical serialization emerged as a challenge to improve the traceability of drugs. It became an urgent necessity in a global effort to combat selling counterfeit medicines, a growing and dangerous phenomenon for patients 'health.

The specific goals are to outline the emerged modern methods to improve the serialization, the existing legislative regulation and the steps forward to global harmonization and the active mechanisms of serialization against counterfeiting medicines. Health care professionals are primarily targeted, along with specialists in the pharmaceutical industry. However, there is a lot of new ground in the area of supply chain management and serialization/ traceability.

The range of counterfeit products reaching markets has also broadened with the increased commercial use of the Internet to provide a dizzying array of both branded and generic drugs. In more than 50% of cases, medicines purchased over the Internet from illegal sites that conceal their physical address have been found to be counterfeit, according to WHO.

"In a shocking development, it was discovered relatively recently that counterfeit versions of lifesaving prescription medicines for cancer and serious cardiovascular diseases are also being sold to consumers online," the European Alliance for Access to Safe Medicines reports.

Developing countries are an obvious target for counterfeiters, because the cost of legitimate drugs may be beyond the reach of much of the population and legal controls are often weak, analysts say.

Counterfeit (or fake) medicines

Counterfeit medicines are medicines which do not respect intellectual property rights and/or violate trademark laws. Counterfeiting can be related to product mislabelling to reproduce an authentic medicine. Another more dangerous method is to supply drugs without or with a lower/higher amount of active pharmaceutical ingredients (API). Also, a serious situation is when medicines contain non-labelled harmful toxic substances.

Fake drugs, as their name tells us, are those counterfeit drugs that are designed to mimic original medicines. Vital drugs such as those for the treatment of malaria, tuberculosis, HIV/AIDS and even anticancer drugs have not escaped forgery

The most common counterfeit drugs

Recently, published data revealed a variety of percentages of falsified drugs based on the geographic areas: 10.5% of medicines are falsified or under dosed, according to WHO worldwide, about 10-30% according to CDC in developing countries versus almost 1% in the U.S. or 13% in Europe industrialized countries. The magnitude of this problem makes it harder to achieve universal access to safe and effective global medicines and the need for further investigation of well-designed prevalence studies are required to reflect the actual prevalence.

In The Beginning: A Brief History

While companies have been discussing the need to identify and verify medicines to protect patient safety for some time, the pharmaceutical industry has been slow to adopt new technologies.

In 1999, following a report by the US institute of Medicine, President Bill Clinton placed patient safety (including preventing errors at the point of dispensing medicines) on the agenda of federal government and continued to lobby for changes after his presidency.

In 2003, the US Food and Drug Administration (FDA) mandated barcoding on unit doses and in the same year, the World Health Organisation (WHO) published a report recognising the scale of the counterfeit medicine challenge stating that 10% of medication worldwide was counterfeit.

A step change took place in serialisation around 2005 and a number of countries began to set deadlines for implementation. However, after making some strides towards securing the supply chain, the challenge became less of a priority during the financial crisis in 2008.

As the global economy has improved, slowly the momentum has shifted. Turkey introduced serialisation requirements in 2010 and other markets such as China, South Korea and India have regulations in place. With the EU Falsified Medicines Directive (FMD) came into effect in February 2019 and the US introduced legislation in November 2017, as part of the Drug Supply Chain Security Act (DSCSA), it's expected that more than 75%

of global medicines will be covered by some form of track and trace regulations by 2019.

While the EU FMD is limited to the verification of medicines at the dispensing point and, therefore, does not allow for the tracing of drug products throughout the whole pharmaceutical supply chain, it is a positive step towards establishing a more secure system.

Basic Concept Of Track And Trace System

Why is Track & Trace becoming increasingly important for businesses?

Product piracy is an increasing problem for businesses in the broadest range of industries. A growing number of companies are forced to confront piracy with measures such as serialization and Tracking & Tracing. Results from surveys show that nearly every second consumer considers counterfeiting as a serious problem, and nearly the same amount reported falling victim to counterfeiting. However, Track & Trace offers businesses far more than assurances against counterfeiting and piracy. The decision to serialize and track products on item level opens up a whole new range of options and can provide real value added for the business. For example, the transparency that is gained as a result can facilitate better control of recalls, loss reduction and the optimization of supply chain, marketing and sales strategies.

What does Track & Trace mean?

'**Tracking**' means monitoring forward movement of finished goods through the supply chain and ensuring that all taxes and duties have been paid and volumes verified (i.e., manufacturer to end user).

'Tracing' means working backwards through the supply chain to establish where any genuine product was diverted out of the legitimate supply chain (i.e., end user to manufacturer for history, recall etc.)

Tracking & Tracing: Provide visibility to specific information (e.g., batch, lot, date, origin, ingredients, safety, or recall status).

why is this useful?

The information can quickly tell the person querying the package or product on: what it is, where it came from, whether it is subject to a recall or other security issue, when and where it was packed or manufactured and in some cases, where the product was supposed to be shipped to (and therefore, whether it's in the correct location).

From serialization over aggregation to Track & Trace

To achieve full Track & Trace the typical approach is to start with serialization. Serialization means to make each single product unique by placing an item identifier on every single product. Typically, the item identifier is a Data Matrix-Code containing at least the product related GTIN paired with a serial number. This way the product becomes the vehicle for carrying the information needed for Track and Trace and can be identified individually. It is also then possible to store further product related information in a database linked to this unique ID. Serialization takes place directly at the production lines and requires in most cases new printing and scanning technologies and software.

The next big step after serialization is achieved is typically the aggregation. Aggregation is the process of building packaging hierarchies and storing this relationship in a database. If, for example single products get packed in a carton and these cartons get packed on a pallet, this relationship has to be recognized and stored in a database using scanning processes. Each new packing level, e.g., cartons or pallets, also requires a unique (serialized) identifier. Aggregation is a major step towards Track & Trace and the big advantage is that; once the packaging hierarchy is built and stored in a database, only the highest-level identifier (e.g., pallet) has to be scanned (identified) and all associated packed items in the hierarchy will automatically be known. This makes it much easier to follow the items through the supply chain, as not every single item needs to be scanned at different intervals in the supply chain. Aggregation can take place directly at production/packaging lines or, for example, in distribution centres during re-packing. In most instances new or additional scanning technology and software is required to capture the building of hierarchies and the movement of product through the supply chain.

Once serialization and aggregation are achieved, everything is in place in order to completely Track & Trace products through the supply chain. The final step is to define points in the supply chain where the products or, the highest packaging level (due to aggregation) has to be scanned. As a result, the state (e.g., produced, shipped, packed, dispensed, etc.) of all packed items can be changed in the database where the Track & Trace data is stored (e.g., EPCIS). While serialization and aggregation take place in production and packaging lines or in distribution centers, Tracking & Tracing mostly takes place in the supply chain.

The combination of having a unique identifier and capturing the information relating to the movement of these aggregated products (when, where, what and why) is the best way to achieve a safe, secure and transparent supply chain.

How does Track & Trace work?

The key to implement Track & Trace is the ability to put variable data on item, case and/or pallet level (depending on the granularity to which items need to be tracked) and to trace these items through the supply chain. Radio-frequency identification and barcodes are two common technology methods used to deliver traceability.

Typically, a barcode or RFID transponder usually containing a combination of GTIN and serial number will be applied to items on the production line. In some cases, there will be an aggregation of the products, related to the packaging hierarchy (e.g., item to case and case to pallet). Aggregation makes it easier to trace a bundle of items through the supply chain as only the ID of the pallet has to be scanned and therefore identifying all cases and items contained on the pallet.

Once the IDs are applied to the products; all product related events such as 'produced', 'shipped', 'received', 'dispensed' will be captured along the supply chain via scanning of these IDs with mobile devices. This captured information will be stored in a database (EPCIS) together with product related information from production such as 'batch', 'manufacturing date', 'expiration date' etc.

Why traceability?

Traceability can help in providing the visibility and intelligence of both global market opportunity as well as risk, in an effective and speedy manner. Speed and availability of data is often a necessity to mitigate risk and to identify and exploit new opportunities.

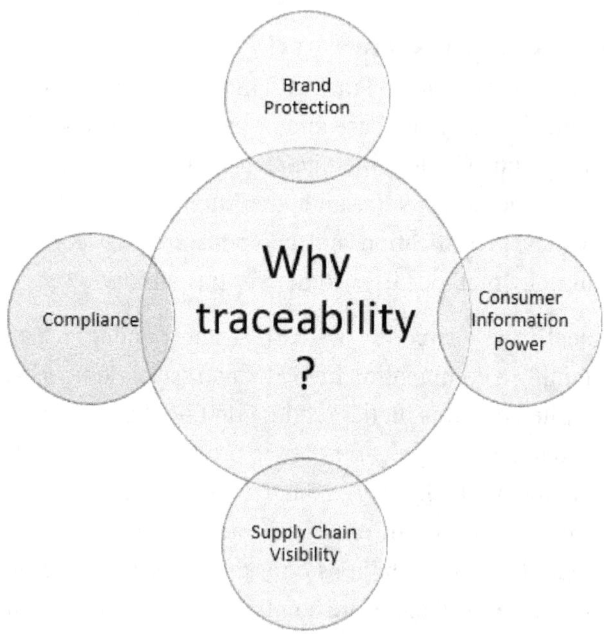

Different ways of Traceability

Track and Trace or Tracking and Tracing, concerns a process of determining the current and past locations (and other information) of a unique item or property.

Traceability Types

when looking at traceability one can distinguish different types of traceability

- **Traceability of a product genealogy**
  - ✓ Batch- or serial number component level

- **Product supply chain traceability**
  - ✓ Serialized
  - ✓ Item serialized.
  - ✓ Batch level
  - ✓ GTIN or part number level

- **Product provenance and pedigree**
- **Logistical Track & Trace**
  - ✓ Parcel traceability
  - ✓ Sea-freight container traceability
  - ✓ Pallet level traceability

- **Process traceability**
  - ✓ Procure-to-pay or order-to-cash

- **Traceability for sustainability and product footprint data recording**

Importance Of Track And Trace System

Increasing Productivity

With track and trace systems, there is an environment that supports competition for drug manufacturers. With the information obtained by the systems, it is possible to carry out studies that will increase sales and productivity in pharmaceutical production.

Ensuring Serialization and Traceability

In the US and EU, Companies have gone one step further than serialization and have started to develop track and trace solutions using Data Matrix, RFID and QR code. Drug flow between production and sales channels can be monitored with these systems. All the manufacturers have to implement some kind of track and trace solution to their production line until the 2019.

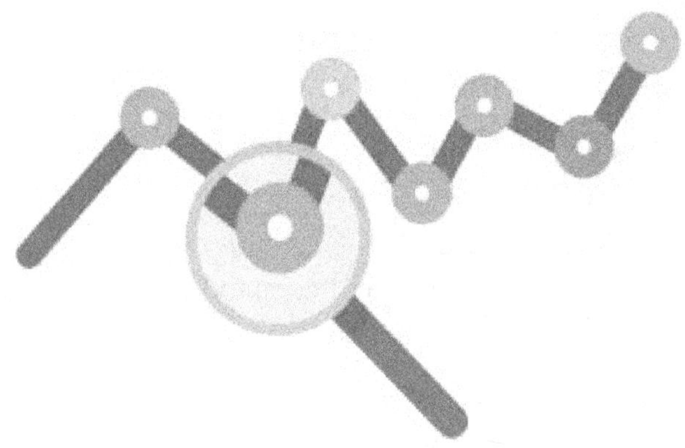

War with the Counterfeit and Illicit Drugs

Drug manufacturers cannot fight the counterfeit and illicit drugs alone. With investments of government and companies in track and trace solutions, counterfeit and illicit drugs can be identified. Market penetration of counterfeit drugs will be prevented from the beginning.

Although drug track and trace systems have been able to provide traceability and increase productivity with the information registered in these systems, they have not been able to be used everywhere in the world because of the obstacles that are present today.

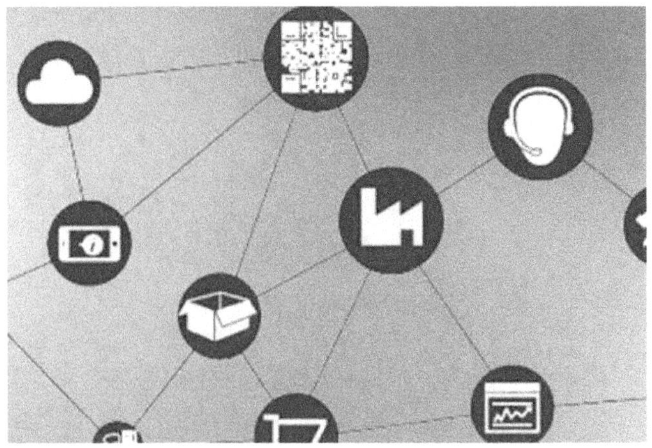

Obstacles

No Common Standards

At the very least, the inability to establish a national standard is the greatest obstacle to serialization and the implementation of drug track and trace solutions.

In the US, the Food and Drug Administration (FDA) has asked the pharmaceutical industry to set a general standard for track and trace all drugs. The idea of establishing a common standard has arisen from the desire to assemble all the industry leaders under a common roof, facilitating their adaptation.

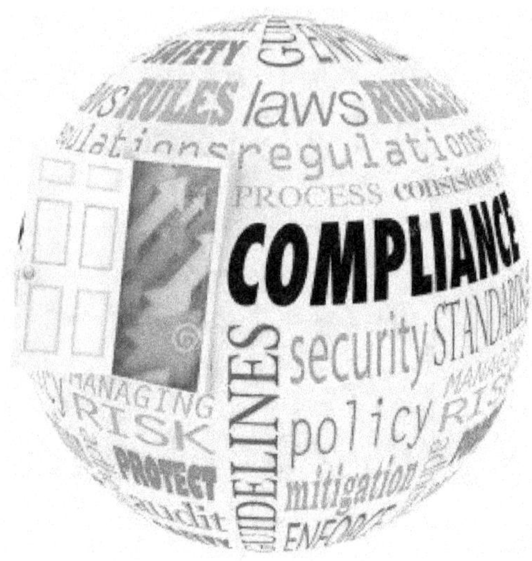

Safety Concerns

Some drug companies argue that the barcode system is not secure and is easily changeable. Apart from this, due to the presence of important personal information, there is concern that the track and trace system will be used by unauthorized people to access the information.

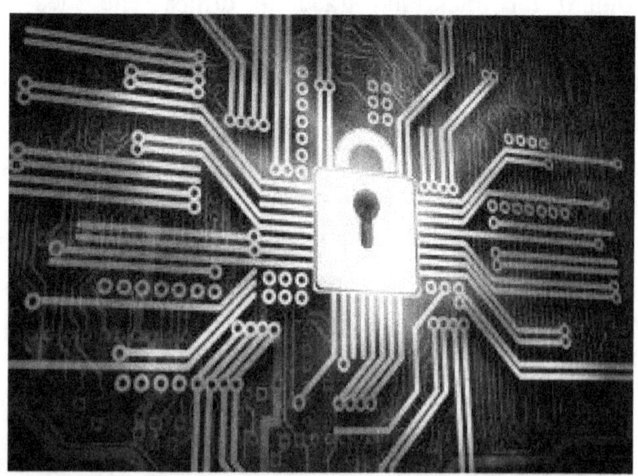

Slowing the Production Lines

Manufacturer thinks that the barcoding systems which is a part of the track and trace system, will slow down the production line and have increasing costs. This belief has made the implementation process difficult.

To resolve these concerns, track and trace systems should be studied in detail and every country should establish their standards according to their processes.

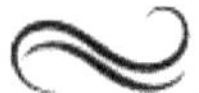

Chapter | 2

Pharma Serialization System

Pharma Serialization – The Most Comprehensive Description

Governments have developed an effective and efficient method of combating drug counterfeiting that directly affects public health in the last decade. The main goal of this method is that we can trace the drug during the supply process. The first step to implement the method is pharma serialization.

Serialisation in the pharmaceutical industry is one of the best tools society has to combat counterfeit medicines.

Counterfeit medicines are a risk to public health. They are often not effective so don't benefit patients. If that is not dangerous enough, counterfeit drugs can also actively harm patients, even causing death.

Counterfeit drugs also damage the pharmaceutical industry. They directly cause lost revenues plus they can have knock-on effects including unwarranted reputational damage, loss of patient confidence, and more.

Over the past decade, many legislators have prepared laws and regulations that make pharma serialization obligatory. DSCSA in the United States, EU-FMD in the European Union, and ITS in Turkey are the most notable examples. Pharmaceutical manufacturers and other players in the industry face problems from time to time as they try to assure compliance with the requirements of these regulations.

What Is Pharma Serialization?

Pharma Serialization is assigning a unique code to the packaging of each drug and printing this code on the packaging by any method. There are two main points in this definition. The first is the unique code and the second is the drug packaging.

The definition and structure of the unique code are defined within the regulations of the countries. The unique code definition within the regulations of all countries is largely similar to each other and follows GS1 standards. The areas that differ are generally the codes and cryptography preferences of the reimbursement institutions. In the following table, you can find unique code examples for countries' pharma serialization practices.

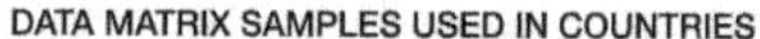

Packaging in the pharmaceutical industry has three main headings.

Primary Packaging: Primary packaging is the packaging in contact with the drug. The aluminium blister is the most common primary packaging used in the vial and bottle industry. The serialization of the primary packaging is not a requirement in any market other than the American and Indian markets. Because only in these markets, even if it is exceptional, the patient can purchase the primary packaging.

Secondary Packaging: It is the packaging that contains the primary packaged medicine or medicines. The best example of this packaging is the carton. On average, 80% of the medicines in the world are sold in a carton. The serialization of this packaging is a must for regulations compliance. Some regulations, such as EU-FMD, require Tamper Evident, along with pharma serialization, to guarantee that the medicine is first opened by the patient.

Tertiary Packaging: You can carry out B2B operations in the supply chain by making medicines into a whole with tertiary packaging. The best examples of tertiary packaging are bundles, cases, and pallets. The serialization of tertiary packaging is the most important point to ensure traceability in the supply chain.

Pharma Serialisation Process:

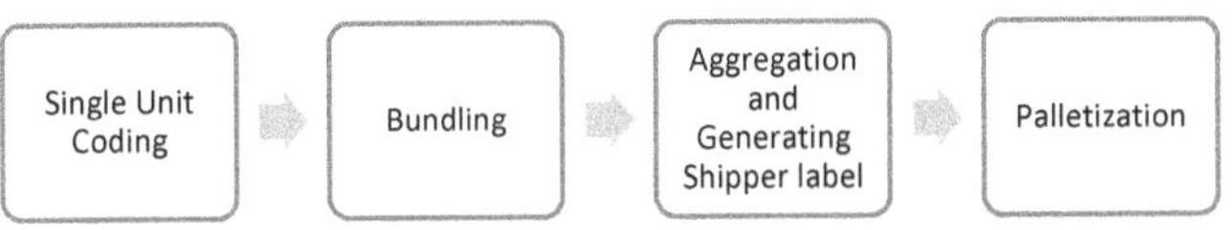

Challenges In Serialization Faced By Pharmaceutical Companies

Like any other change across the supply chain, serialization has its own set of challenges for the pharmaceutical companies. Here is a look into some of the potential challenging areas when it comes to implementing serialization:

Hardware Setup and Updates: Companies will need to make sure they have highly functioning hardware to manufacture labels, barcodes, and seals that are essential for serialization.

Label redesign: For many manufacturers, serialization will require a significant redesign of labels to allow space for the new 2D barcode. Consequently, changes in labelling may also necessitate alterations or redesign of packaging structure or graphic elements.

Steady Flow of the Production Line: Sticking to the process of serialization and making your skill base acquainted with this process might slow down the production line. The use of labels for individual units will also significantly slow down the packaging process.

Overall Cost Inflation: Cost inflation is a given when it comes to serialization, given the costs involved in hardware and software. However, this can be negated via pooled-investments and sustainable applications of the hardware and software.

Skilled Personnel Shortage: Newer, digitized ways of serialization would require a skill base that is well acquainted with the technicalities and details of these techniques. Currently, companies are facing a lack of a skilled employee base that is technically sound enough to implement their serialization strategies seamlessly.

Data management and availability: In addition to physical packaging changes, data management needs will grow rapidly. The IT architecture must be able to generate, store, capture and transmit millions of serial numbers for numerous supply chains.

Assembling a cross-functional team: Serialization has both information and production-floor aspects. Experts from IT, processing/packaging, engineering, labelling, quality assurance and project management must cooperate to ensure a smooth implementation.

Technical Glitches: Serialization is a process that requires minimal human intervention, and while that can be beneficial to avoid manual error, there is also a possibility of technical glitches in the process leading to incorrect tagging and compromised track and trace.

Key Benefits Of Serialization Implementation

- End-to-end implementation across the supply chain for drugs in a hassle-free way

- Seamlessly sealing the supply chain loopholes to combat drug counterfeiting and warehouse packaging glitches.

- Minimal human intervention needed, making serialization a full-proof, effective way to ensure brand authenticity and mitigate batch recalls.

- Total compliance with the traceability regulations.

- serialization will lead to increased transparency and visibility by reducing counterfeiting, diversion and theft.

- The ability to trace product locations, supply chain partners can increase shipping accuracy and more quickly remove recalled and defective products.

Pharma Serialization Reconciliation

The purpose of the pharmaceutical reconciliation process is to ensure that all materials used for finished products have been correctly accounted for and no errors have occurred. The reconciliation helps to avoid releasing a non-conforming product and is the very foundation for ensuring product integrity in the product supply chain and, ultimately, patient safety.

However, pharmaceutical finished goods manufacturing is already changing extensively due to global serialisation and traceability regulations. These regulations require that each and every medicine sales package requires unique numbering and traceability throughout the supply chain – right up to the patients. Obviously, implementing these new capabilities in the finished pharma manufacturing should help improve the medicinal product's integrity and comply with the current reconciliation requirements specified in the regulatory GxP (Good Practices) guidelines, especially by the US Food and Drug Administration (FDA) and European Medicines Agency (EMA).

Pharma serialisation reconciliation ensures that the serial numbers are used correctly for finished products with traceability in each phase of the pharmaceutical packaging process; beginning with the creation of serial numbers, and ending with supplying the finished serialised products to the market.

Pharma serialisation reconciliation process

The serialisation reconciliation process can be divided into three phases based on the batch packaging execution process (lot):

1. **Pre-lot reconciliation** for the reservation, creation, and provision of serial numbers to the packaging lines. The pre-lot phase defines the total amount of available serial numbers used for the packaging.

2. **In-lot reconciliation** covers the serial number usage for finished products and shipping cases/pallets (aggregation), as well as in-line disposal and quality management sampling. The in-lot phase defines the actual serial number consumption in the packaging. In addition, EMVS (European Medicines Verification Service) reporting needs to be done as part of the in-lot reconciliation.

3. **Post-lot reconciliation** covers the changes with the serialized products and aggregation after packaging completion but prior to the change of custody, e.g., warehouse damage control and quality control sampling.

Pre-lot reconciliation: getting ready for the serialization.

If required, the yield for the pre-lot reconciled serial numbers can be calculated as follows:

$$Yield_{Pre-lot} = \frac{Allocated\ Serial\ Numbers}{Total\ Serial\ Numbers} * 100$$

Allocated serial numbers is basically the total planned lot size.

Total serial numbers is the number of serial numbers reserved for the lot.

In-lot reconciliation: ensuring compliance.

The in-lot reconciliation is obviously the most important phase from the quality management and GMP compliance point of view.

If required, the yield for the in-lot reconciled serial numbers can be calculated as follows:

$$Yield_{In-lot} = \frac{Activated + Damaged + Destroyed + QA\ Sampled\ Serial\ Numbers}{Allocated\ Serial\ Numbers} * 100$$

The in-lot serial number changes are recorded either in the serialisation vendor plant, or site server, or in the manufacturer's centralised serialisation repository.

Post-lot reconciliation: supplying products to the market

The post-lot reconciliation covers the changes that occur after the packaging stage, but while the serialised products are still in the manufacturer's custody – e.g., in staging, transit and warehouse.

However, any such changes need to be recorded and potentially also reported to MAHs and regulators.

If required, the yield for the post-lot reconciliation can be calculated as follows:

$$Yield_{Post-lot} = \frac{Activated\ Serial\ Numbers - (Damaged + Destroyed + QA\ Sampled)}{Activated\ Serial\ Numbers} * 100$$

For the highest-level reconciliation accuracy and supply network manageability, it is highly recommended to use aggregation. This ensures more cost-efficient supply network operations and traceability on a case and pallet level.

Serialization Solutions Levels

What does the "L" stand for in L1-L5 solution provider?

The "L" in "L1-L5 solution provider" stands for "level," as in the level of serialization in a supply chain. To put a finer point on it, it means the level of serialization and information management in a supply chain. And if you hadn't guessed, there are five levels:

Level 1: Device

Level 2: Packaging

Level 3: Site

Level 4: Enterprise

Level 5: Network

The list above progresses from the smallest or most localized level, the L1 device level, to the most expansive and all-encompassing level, the L5 network level. Generally, L1, L2, and L3 are grouped together because they're happening where products are created and packaged; L4 and L5 are paired together in the realm where those products enter the greater supply chain to make their way to their final destinations.

When talking about L1-L5, let's work backwards from largest to smallest. This way, we can "zoom in on" the details and put everything in a more vivid context.

Level 5: Network

L5 is where has its roots and where we built our reputation for supply chain excellence. The network level is where all serialization and regulatory data is managed, including with your trading partners, regulatory authorities and their repositories, and customers. It ensures you're communicating with partners and complying with regulations.

Level 4: Enterprise

which manages and verifies all your serialization and regulatory data/compliance reporting before sending it to L5. It also generates your serial numbers and manages all your business processes. When you design your solutions for L1, L2, and L3, you must decide how they will integrate with your L4 solution.

Level 3: Site

This is where we enter your actual manufacturing facilities and processes. L3 manages the line systems (i.e., L2) at your site to ensure that they are working optimally. L3 is optional; if present, it serves as the "middle man" between L4 and L2, requesting serial numbers from the former and allocating them to the latter. L3 will also verify the L2 data before it is submitted to L4.

Level 2: Packaging

L2 systems control the L1 hardware and manage the serial numbers which are printed and applied on packages by L1 devices. L2 systems will communicate with the L4 (or L3, f present) to send/receive serial numbers as needed.

Level 1: Device

L1 comprises devices on a packaging line that enable serial numbers to be affixed to packaging and products, such as barcode printers, label printers, and labellers. It also includes cameras and scanners used for quality control, such as visual inspections of products and labelling.

What Is Aggregation?

Aggregation can be a part of the serialisation solution on your production lines. Serialisation involves adding a unique identifier to each product at individual pack level, i.e. at the level patients or customers receive the product.

> *"If you are designing a track and trace system for a product sold in high quantities, your process will become chaotic without pharmaceutical aggregation".*

However, those individual pack-level products do not get from the production line to the patient/customer through the distribution chain as an individual pack-level product. Instead, multiple individual pack level products are packed in cases and then multiple cases are packed on pallets.

An aggregation solution adds codes to the outside of cases and pallets to identify the individual pack-level products inside. In other words, aggregation builds parent-child relationships from pallet to case to individual pack-level products.

This makes it possible to find out what is inside a case or pallet by scanning the code on the outside, i.e., you don't need to open the case to get the serial number of each individual pack-level product.

Aggregation is the process of building a data relationship between unique identifiers for saleable units, the cartons they are packed into, and then the cases and pallets into which they are subsequently packed and shipped. Using that data, manufacturer distribution operations can "infer" that the correct product and quantity are enclosed in each carton, case, or pallet without opening each for inspection.

Pharmaceutical serialisation process:

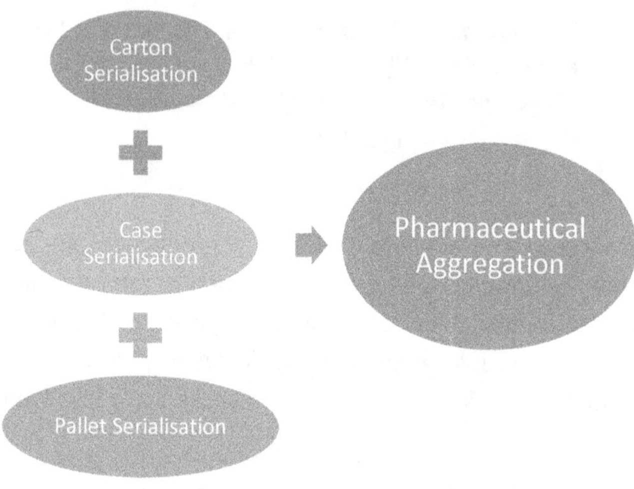

*"Aggregation is not mandatory everywhere yet. However, **we have decided to anticipate future regulations**. For example, we have integrated aggregation into our processes which is an important strategic choice that is part of our long-term strategy and development".*

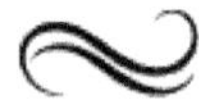

Chapter | 3

Global Standards Behind Serializations And Traceability

For the last 30 years, GS1 has been dedicated to the design and implementation of global standards for use in the supply chain. GS1 standards provide a framework that allows products, services, and information about them to move efficiently and securely for the benefit of businesses and the improvement of people's lives, every day, everywhere.

> *"GS1 designs and manages a global system of supply chain standards".*

GS1 standards bring together companies representing all parts of the supply chain – manufacturers, distributors, retailers, hospitals, transporters, customs organisations, software developers, local and international regulatory authorities, and more.

Perhaps you are an expert on retail supply chain standards; perhaps you are involved in deploying an automatic identification project in the healthcare sector;

or a traceability programme in the field of transport and logistics. Or perhaps you're not so closely involved with that aspect of your business or your industry.

In short, well-designed standards allow organisations to focus on how to use information rather than how to get information.

> *"Companies care about the value and the benefits that standards bring".*

The GS1 System of Standards is a much better choice, however, because it is global, robust, multi-sector, user generated, and scalable.

Global: The GS1 System of Standards is truly global.

Robust: GS1 Communication Standards have benefited from multiple data accuracy improvements; and together the GS1 System is solid and scalable.

Multi-sector: the GS1 System of Standards has been endorsed by a wide variety of industries.

User-generated: All GS1 standards are built and maintained through the GS1 Global Standards Management Process (GSMP), a worldwide collaborative forum.

Scalable: Whether you are a small company or a large one, whether you have one single product or hundreds, the GS1 System of Standards is perfectly suited to your needs.

> ***The GS1 System of Standards is global, robust, multi-sector, user-generated, and scalable, and it is used today by millions of companies across dozens of industry sectors.***

The GS1 System of Standards is a flexible architecture that ensures maximum efficiency. It is built around and upon two main elements: GS1 Automatic Identification Standards and GS1 Communication Standards. GS1 Automatic Identification Standards are themselves composed of several elements: GS1 Identification (ID) Keys and Application Identifiers, GS1 Data Carriers and the EPC Identifier.

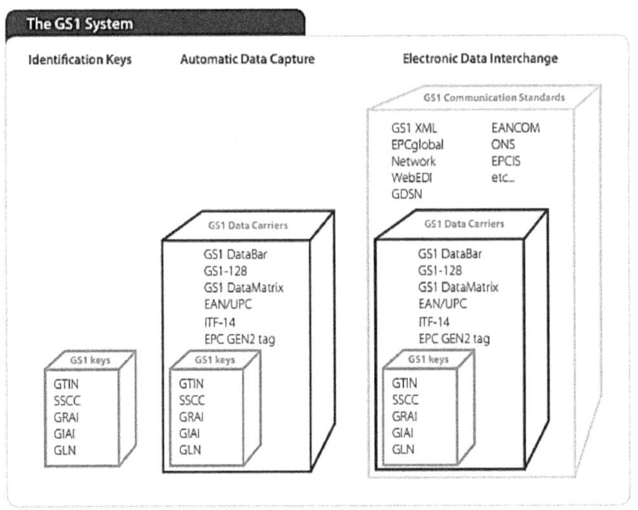

How GS1 Standards Work

Identify

GS1 identification standards include standards that define unique identification codes (called GS1 identification keys) which may be used by an information system to refer unambiguously to a real-world entity such as a:

- trade item
- logistics unit
- physical location
- document
- service relationship
- other entity

Capture

GS1 data capture standards currently include definitions of bar code and radio-frequency identification (RFID) data carriers which allow GS1 Identification Keys and supplementary data to be affixed directly to a physical object, and standards that specify consistent interfaces to readers, printers, and other hardware and software components that connect the data carriers to business applications.

Share

GS1 standards for information sharing include data standards for master data, business transaction data, and physical event data, as well as communication standards for sharing this data between applications and trading partners. Other information sharing standards include discovery standards that help locate where relevant data resides across a supply chain and trust standards that help establish the conditions for sharing data with adequate security.

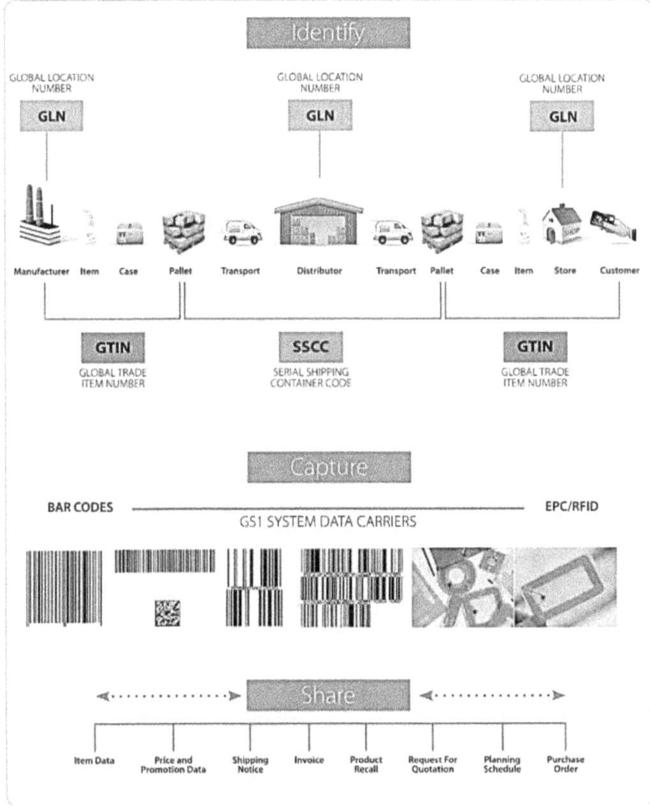

GS1 Automatic Identification

- GS1 Identification Keys & Application Identifiers
- GS1 Data Carriers
- The Electronic Product Code (EPC)

GS1 Identification Keys are used to name and distinguish any object, thing, or location, so interested parties can get information or business messages related to them.

The main GS1 ID keys are:
- Global Trade Item Number (GTIN)
- Global Location Number (GLN)
- Serial Shipping Container Code (SSCC)

Other GS1 ID Keys
- Global Returnable Asset Identifier (GRAI)
- Global Individual Asset Identifier (GIAI)
- Global Service Relation Number (GSRN)
- Global Document Type Identifier (GDTI)
- Global Shipment Identification Number (GSIN)
- Global Identification Number for Consignment (GINC)
- Global Coupon Number (GCN)
- Component/Part Identifier (CPID)
- Global Model Number (GMN)

Global Trade Item Number (GTIN)

The GS1 Key for unique product identification is the Global Trade Item Number (GTIN) which is assigned AI (01). GTINs are used to identify "trade items" (i.e., products and services that may be priced, ordered or invoiced at any point in the supply chain). They are assigned by the responsible entity who is normally responsible for the allocation of the GTIN.

> *The GTIN is used to uniquely identify trade items.*
> *Each trade item that is different from another is*
> *allocated its own separate GTIN.*

GTINs provide accuracy, speed and efficiencies to millions of companies around the world, in all areas of modern business.

There is also a serialised form of the GTIN: a Serialised GTIN identifies the specific instance of a trade item. For example, serialised GTINs are used in the healthcare sector to distinguish individual implants which are otherwise of the same brand and characteristics; or in tyre production to differentiate individual tyres so that they can be tracked through their lifecycle. Serialised GTINs, for example, enable tyres on commercial lorries to be maintained at proper intervals and withdrawn from use when they have been in circulation a certain amount of time.

Overview of GTIN formats

	GS1 Company Prefix									Item reference			Check digit
(GTIN-13)		N_1	N_2	N_3	N_4	N_5	N_6	N_7	N_8	N_9	N_{10}	N_{11}	N_{12}	N_{13}
(GTIN-14)	N_1	N_2	N_3	N_4	N_5	N_6	N_7	N_8	N_9	N_{10}	N_{11}	N_{12}	N_{13}	N_{14}
	U.P.C. Company Prefix									Item reference			Check digit
(GTIN-12)			N_1	N_2	N_3	N_4	N_5	N_6	N_7	N_8	N_9	N_{10}	N_{11}	N_{12}
						GS1-8 Prefix				Item reference			Check digit
(GTIN-8)							N_1	N_2	N_3	N_4	N_5	N_6	N_7	N_8

Anatomy Of A GTIN-14

There are four components that make up a GTIN-14.

1. Indicator Digit

2. GS1 Company Prefix (GCP)

3. Item Reference

4. Check Digit

1	2	3	4	5	6	7	8	9	10	11	12	13	14
Ind	GS1 Company Prefix						Item Reference						Chk
1	0	3	0	4	0	9	4	9	2	1	3	4	8

GLN - Global Location Number

The Global Location Number, or GLN, is the GS1 ID Key used to identify locations and legal entities.

Locations can be a physical place such as a warehouse, a storage cabinet or even a specific shelf within a store; they can be a legal entity such as a company, or division of a company; or they can be a function that takes place within a legal entity, such as the accounting department of a company or the paediatrics ward of a hospital.

GLNs are also the essential building block for a variety of EPC/RFID applications built around event capture.

> ***The GLN identifies any location anywhere in the world in a unique way.***

GLN in electronic data sharing standards The GLN is widely used in the sharing of electronic data between companies, since it enables unambiguous identification of the parties, locations and systems. Therefore, the GLN is a foundational key in the related GS1 standards.

EDI Electronic Data Interchange (EDI) ideally uses Global Location Numbers (GLNs) to identify all trading partners and physical locations involved. Also, the EDI mailbox or network address for companies is often identified with a GLN. The EDI standards promoted by the GS1 system (EANCOM, GS1 XML) make full use of GLNs to simplify the automation of business messaging.

GDSN Data pools and the GS1 Global Registry that links them for the purpose of global data synchronisation mandate the use of GLNs to identify each party that provides information to any data pool or who requires information about products and locations.

The GLN is a multi-sector global solution for identifying locations at whatever level of granularity is needed. This ISO-compliant identifier removes the need for complicated proprietary location numbering systems. Its global uniqueness is guaranteed by its structure:

GLN – Global Location Number

Global Location Number Structure		
GS1 Company Prefix	Location Reference	Check Digit
N_1 N_2 N_3 N_4 N_5 N_6 N_7 N_8 N_9 N_{10} N_{11} N_{12}		N_{13}

a. **GS1 Prefix:** Provides a number capacity to each GS1 Member Organisation and enables local administration.

b. **Company number:** Combined with the GS1 Prefix this forms the GS1 Company Prefix allowing companies to allocate GTIN and other GS1 ID Keys

c. **Item Reference:** Allocated by the company with each different product receiving a different number **d. Check Digit:** Calculated from all other digits to provide extra security.

SSCC – Serial Shipping Container Code

The Serial Shipping Container Code (SSCC) is the GS1 ID Key used to identify individual logistic units.

A logistic unit can be any combination of units put together in a carton, in a case, on a pallet or on a truck, where the specific unit load needs to be managed through the supply chain. The SSCC enables a unit to be tracked individually, providing benefits for order and delivery tracking and automated goods-receiving.

> *The SSCC identifies individual logistic units, like cartons, crates, or pallets.*

As the SSCC provides a unique number, it can also be utilised as a look-up number to provide not only detailed information regarding the contents of the load, but also as part of an Advanced Shipping Notice (ASN) or Despatch Advice process. Furthermore, with an SSCC, a company can reliably look up details about complex loads, which saves the sender from having to encode long consignment information on individual logistic unit labels.

The SSCC links barcode or EPC/RFID tag information to electronic communications about the logistic unit. SSCCs are ISO licence plate-compliant (ISO/IEC 15459) for tracking and tracing logistic units. Its structure:

a. **GS1 Application Identifier:** provides the meaning of the data field which follows, allowing the same GS1 Data Carrier to encode multiple data.

b. **Extension Digit:** allocated by the user to increase capacity.

c. **GS1 Company Prefix:** Allocated by GS1 Member Organisations to member companies enabling them to allocate SSCCs.

d. **Serial Reference:** Allocated by the creator of the logistic unit with each logistic unit receiving a different number.

e. **Check Digit:** Calculated from all other digits to provide extra security.

Other GS1 ID Keys

GSRN – Global Service Relation Number: The Global Service Relation Number is the GS1 ID Key used to identify a service relationship between a business and a client, such as club membership, loyalty programmes, or a patient in a hospital.

GRAI – Global Returnable Asset Identifier: The Global Returnable Asset Identifier (GRAI) is one of the two GS1 ID Keys for asset identification. As its name indicates, the GRAI is used to identify returnable assets.

The GRAI can be used simply for asset identification and tracking purposes, or it can be part of a hiring or rental system where two or more companies collaborate, as it allows enterprises to scan assets into and out of their businesses.

GIAI – Global Individual Asset Identifier: The Global Individual Asset Identifier (GIAI) is the second of two GS1 ID Keys for asset identification. GIAIs are used to identify fixed assets of any value within a company that need to be identified uniquely, such as a computer, a desk, a vehicle or a component part. Having a unique identifier for their assets allows a business to identify, track and manage them across their entire life.

GDTI – Global Document Type Identifier: The Global Document Type Identifier (GDTI) is the GS1 ID Key to identify a document by type. The term "document" here is applied broadly to cover any official or private papers that infer a right (e.g., a proof of ownership) or an obligation (e.g., call for military service) upon the bearer. Other examples of the kinds of documents that could have a GDTI are tax demands, proof of shipment forms, insurance policies, internal invoices, nationalised or standardised exams, and passports.

GSIN – Global Shipment Identification Number: The Global Shipment Identification Number (bill of lading) is a number assigned by a seller (sender) of the goods. It provides a globally unique number that identifies a logical grouping of physical units for the purpose of a transport shipment.

GINC – Global Identification Number for Consignment: The Global Identification Number for Consignment identifies a logical grouping of goods (one or more physical entities) that has been consigned to a freight forwarder or carrier and is intended to be transported as a whole.

GS1 Application Identifiers

The GS1 ID Keys are complemented by the GS1 Application Identifiers (or GS1 AIs).

GS1 AIs act like a code list of generic and simple data fields for use in multi-sector and international supply chain applications. Each GS1 AI consists of two or more digits and provides the definition, format and structure of the data field encoded in a GS1 Data Carrier. For example, a GS1 AI exists for each GS1 ID Key, allowing it to be encoded in GS1 Barcodes or EPC/RFID tags.

> **"GS1 AIs present a standardised way to encode information in a single GS1 Data Carrier".**

GS1 Application Identifiers

AI	Data Content	Format [1]	FNC1 required [4]	Data title
00	*Identification of a logistic unit (SSCC): AI (00)*	N2+N18		SSCC
01	*Identification of a trade item (GTIN): AI (01)*	N2+N14		GTIN
10	*Batch or lot number: AI (10)*	N2+X..20	(FNC1)	BATCH/LOT
11 [2]	*Production date: AI (11)*	N2+N6		PROD DATE
12 [2]	*Due date for amount on payment slip: AI (12)*	N2+N6		DUE DATE
13 [2]	*Packaging date: AI (13)*	N2+N6		PACK DATE
15 [2]	*Best before date: AI (15)*	N2+N6		BEST BEFORE or BEST BY
16 [2]	*Sell by date: AI (16)*	N2+N6		SELL BY
17 [2]	*Expiration date: AI (17)*	N2+N6		USE BY OR EXPIRY
20	*Internal product variant: AI (20)*	N2+N2		VARIANT
21	*Serial number: AI (21)*	N2+X..20	(FNC1)	SERIAL

240	*Additional product identification assigned by the manufacturer: AI (240)*	N3+X..30	(FNC1)	ADDITIONAL ID
250	*Secondary serial number: AI (250)*	N3+X..30	(FNC1)	SECONDARY SERIAL
253	*Global Document Type Identifier (GDTI): AI (253)*	N3+N13+X..17	(FNC1)	GDTI
254	*Global Location Number (GLN) extension component: AI (254)*	N3+X..20	(FNC1)	GLN EXTENSION COMPONENT
255	*Global Coupon Number (GCN): AI (255)*	N3+N13+N..12	(FNC1)	GCN
30	*Variable count of items: AI (30)*	N2+N..8	(FNC1)	VAR. COUNT
37	*Count of trade items or trade item pieces contained in a logistic unit: AI (37)*	N2+N..8	(FNC1)	COUNT
390n [3]	*Amount payable or coupon value - Single monetary area: AI (390n)*	N4+N..15	(FNC1)	AMOUNT
400	*Customer's purchase order number: AI (400)*	N3+X..30	(FNC1)	ORDER NUMBER
401	*Global Identification Number for Consignment (GINC): AI (401)*	N3+X..30	(FNC1)	GINC
402	*Global Shipment Identification Number (GSIN): AI (402)*	N3+N17	(FNC1)	GSIN
403	*Routing code: AI (403)*	N3+X..30	(FNC1)	ROUTE
410	*Ship to - Deliver to Global Location Number (GLN): AI (410)*	N3+N13		SHIP TO LOC

411	*Bill to - Invoice to Global Location Number (GLN): AI (411)*	N3+N13		BILL TO
412	*Purchased from Global Location Number (GLN): AI (412)*	N3+N13		PURCHASE FROM
413	*Ship for - Deliver for - Forward to Global Location Number (GLN): AI (413)*	N3+N13		SHIP FOR LOC
414	*Identification of a physical location - Global Location Number (GLN): AI (414)*	N3+N13		LOC No
415	*Global Location Number (GLN) of the invoicing party: AI (415)*	N3+N13		PAY TO
416	*Global Location Number (GLN) of the production or service location: AI (416)*	N3+N13		PROD/SERV LOC
417	*Party Global Location Number (GLN): AI (417)*	N3+N13		PARTY
420	*Ship-to / Deliver-to postal code within a single postal authority: AI (420)*	N3+X..20	(FNC1)	SHIP TO POST
421	*Ship-to / Deliver-to postal code with three-digit ISO country code: AI (421)*	N3+N3+X..9	(FNC1)	SHIP TO POST

AI	Data Content	Format [1]	FNC1 required [4]	Data title
422	*Country of origin of a trade item: AI (422)*	N3+N3	(FNC1)	ORIGIN
423	*Country of initial processing: AI (423)*	N3+N3+N..12	(FNC1)	COUNTRY - INITIAL PROCESS.
424	*Country of processing: AI (424)*	N3+N3	(FNC1)	COUNTRY - PROCESS.
425	*Country of disassembly: AI (425)*	N3+N3+N..12	(FNC1)	COUNTRY - DISASSEMBLY
426	*Country covering full process chain: AI (426)*	N3+N3	(FNC1)	COUNTRY – FULL PROCESS
427	*Country subdivision of origin code for a trade item: AI (427)*	N3+X..3	(FNC1)	ORIGIN SUBDIVISION
4300	*Ship-to / Deliver-to Company name: AI (4300)*	N4+X..35	(FNC1)	SHIP TO COMP
4301	*Ship-to / Deliver-to contact name: AI (4301)*	N4+X..35	(FNC1)	SHIP TO NAME
4302	*Ship-to / Deliver-to address line 1: AI (4302)*	N4+X..70	(FNC1)	SHIP TO ADD1
4303	*Ship-to /*	N4+X..70	(FNC1)	SHIP TO ADD2

	Deliver-to address line 2: AI (4303)			
4304	*Ship-to / Deliver-to suburb: AI (4304)*	N4+X..70	(FNC1)	SHIP TO SUB
4305	*Ship-to / Deliver-to locality: AI (4305)*	N4+X..70	(FNC1)	SHIP TO LOC
4306	*Ship-to / Deliver-to region: AI (4306)*	N4+X..70	(FNC1)	SHIP TO REG
4307	*Ship-to / Deliver-to country code: AI (4307)*	N4+X2	(FNC1)	SHIP TO COUNTRY
4308	*Ship-to / Deliver-to telephone number: AI (4308)*	N4+X..30	(FNC1)	SHIP TO PHONE
4326	*Release date: AI (4326)*	N4+N6	(FNC1)	REL DATE
7001	*NATO Stock Number (NSN): AI (7001)*	N4+N13	(FNC1)	NSN
7003	*Expiration date and time: AI (7003)*	N4+N10	(FNC1)	EXPIRY TIME
7023	*Global Individual Asset Identifier of an assembly: AI (7023)*	N4+X..30	(FNC1)	GIAI – ASSEMBLY
7040	*GS1 UIC with Extension 1 and Importer*	N4+N1+X3	(FNC1)	UIC+EXT

	index: AI (7040)			
710	*National Healthcare Reimbursement Number (NHRN) – Germany PZN: AI (710)*	N3+X..20	(FNC1)	NHRN PZN
711	*National Healthcare Reimbursement Number (NHRN) – France CIP: AI 711)*	N3+X..20	(FNC1)	NHRN CIP
712	*National Healthcare Reimbursement Number (NHRN) – Spain CN: AI (712)*	N3+X..20	(FNC1)	NHRN CN
713	*National Healthcare Reimbursement Number (NHRN) – Brasil DRN: AI (713)*	N3+X..20	(FNC1)	NHRN DRN
714	*National Healthcare Reimbursement Number (NHRN) – Portugal AIM: AI (714)*	N3+X..20	(FNC1)	NHRN AIM
... [5]	*National Healthcare Reimbursement Number (NHRN) –*	N3+X..20	(FNC1)	NHRN xxx

	Country "A" NHRN			
8003	*Global Returnable Asset Identifier (GRAI): AI (8003)*	N4+N14+X..16	(FNC1)	GRAI
8004	*Global Individual Asset Identifier (GIAI): AI (8004)*	N4+X..30	(FNC1)	GIAI
90	*Information mutually agreed between trading partners: AI (90)*	N2+X..30	(FNC1)	INTERNAL
91 to 99	*Company internal information: AIs (91 - 99)*	N2+X..90	(FNC1)	INTERNAL

NOTES:

(1): The first position indicates the length (number of digits) of the GS1 Application Identifier. The following value refers to the format of the data content. The following convention is applied:

n   implied decimal point position

N   numeric digit

X   any character in figure

N3 3 numeric digits, predefined length

X3 3 characters, fixed length

N..3   up to 3 numeric digits

X..3   up to 3 characters in figure

: If only year and month are available, DD must be filled with two zeroes.

> : The fourth digit of this GS1 Application Identifier indicates the number of decimal places (and in that way the implied decimal point position).
>
> Example:
>
> 3100 Net weight in kg without a decimal point
>
> 3102 Net weight in kg with two decimal places
>
> : All GS1 element strings that begin with GS1 Application Identifiers not contained in the predefined table shown in figure SHALL be separated by a separator character unless this element string is the last one to be encoded in the symbol. For details on the separator character.
>
> An example to illustrate future additional National Healthcare Reimbursement Numbers (NHRNs). If additional NHRN AIs are required, a request for a new NHRN AI SHALL be made through GSMP.
>
> The fourth digit of this GS1 Application Identifier indicates the sequence number, allowing for multiple occurrences of the AI.

GS1 Data Carriers

GS1 has an entire portfolio of Data Carriers: different kinds of media that can hold GS1 ID Keys and attribute data. The same content can, in fact, be encoded onto different kinds of carriers, depending on what use will be made of it.

Overview of GS1 barcodes

The GS1 system uses the following data carriers:

The EAN/UPC symbology family of barcodes (UPC-A, UPC-E, EAN-13, and EAN-8 barcodes and the two- and five-digit add-on symbols) can be read omnidirectionally. These symbols must be used for all items that are scanned at the point-of-sale and may be used on other trade items.	 **UPC-A**	 **EAN-13**
ITF-14 (Interleaved 2-of-5) barcodes carry ID numbers only on trade items that are not expected to pass through the point-of-sale. ITF-14 symbols are better suited for direct printing onto corrugated fibreboard.	 **ITF-14 barcode**	
The GS1-128 barcode is a subset of the Code 128 barcode symbology. Its use is exclusively licenced to GS1. This extremely flexible symbology encodes element strings using GS1 Application Identifiers.	 **GS1-128 barcode**	

GS1 DataBar is a family of linear symbologies used within the GS1 system. This family of linear symbologies in most cases implicitly encodes GS1 Application Identifier (01) and in the case of GS1 DataBar Expanded explicitly encodes element strings using GS1 Application Identifiers.	 **GS1 DataBar Omnidirectional barcode**
GS1 Data Matrix implementing ECC 200 error correction is a subset of ISO/IEC 16022 and is the only version that supports GS1 system data structures encoded with GS1 element string syntax, including Function 1 Symbol Character (FNC1). GS1 Data Matrix SHALL be implemented per approved GS1 system application standards, such as those for regulated healthcare retail consumer trade items.	 **GS1 Data Matrix barcode**
GS1 QR Code, is a subset of ISO/IEC 18004. QR Code supports GS1 system data structures encoding with GS1 element string syntax, including Function 1 Symbol Character (FNC1). GS1 QR Code SHALL be implemented per approved GS1 system application standards.	 **GS1 QR Code barcode**

Symbology Identifiers

The symbology identifier is not encoded in the barcode but is generated by the decoder after decoding and is transmitted as a preamble to the data message.

Structure of the symbology identifiers

Character	Description
]	The flag character (which has an ASCII value of 93). This denotes that the two characters following it are Symbol Identifier characters.
C	The code character. This denotes the type of symbology
M	The modifier character. This indicates the mode in which the symbology is used.

Note: If used, the symbology identifier is transmitted as a prefix to the data message.

Symbology identifier (*)	Symbology format	Content
]E0	EAN-13, UPC-A, or UPC-E	13 digits
]E1	Two-digit add-on symbol	2 digits
]E2	Five-digit add-on symbol	5 digits
]E3	EAN-13, UPC-A, or UPC-E with add-on symbol (**)	15 or 18 digits
]E4	EAN-8	8 digits
]I1	ITF-14	14 digits
]C1	GS1-128	Standard AI element strings
]e0	GS1 DataBar	Standard AI element strings
]e1	GS1 Composite	Data packet containing

		the data following an encoded symbol separator character.
]e2	GS1 Composite	Data packet containing the data following an escape mechanism character.
]d2	GS1 DataMatrix	Standard AI element strings
]Q3	GS1 QR Code	Standard AI element strings
]J1	GS1 DotCode	Standard AI element strings
]d1	Data Matrix implementing ECC 200	GS1 Digital Link URI
]Q1	QR Code	GS1 Digital Link URI

(*) Symbology identifiers are case sensitive.

(**) Barcodes with add-on symbols may be considered either as two separate symbols, each of which is transmitted separately with its own symbology identifier, or as a single data packet. The system designer SHALL select one of these methods, but the method using symbology identifier]E3 is preferable for data security.

Linear barcodes - GS1-128 symbology specifications

The GS1-128 barcode has been carefully designed through joint co-operation between GS1 and AIM (Association for Automatic Identification and Mobility). Use of GS1-128 barcodes provides a high degree of security and distinguishes GS1 system element strings from extraneous non-standard barcodes.

GS1-128 symbology characteristics

The characteristics of the GS1-128 symbology are:

Encodable character set: The GS1 system requires that only the subset of ISO/IEC 646 International Reference Version defined in these GS1 General Specifications be used for GS1 Application Identifier (AI) element strings.

GS1-128 barcodes have a special double character start pattern consisting of the appropriate start character and immediately followed by a Function 1 Symbol Character Code (FNC1). The FNC1 adds to the symbol's non-data overhead. The total symbol overhead is 46 modules.

GS1-128 barcode size characteristics:

- The maximum physical length is 165.10 millimetres (6.500 inch) including Quiet Zones.

- The maximum number of data characters in a single symbol is 48.

- For a given length of data, the symbol size is variable between limits in X-dimension to accommodate the ranges in quality achievable by the various printing processes.

GS1-128 barcode structure

The GS1-128 barcode is made up as follows, reading from left to right:

- Left Quiet Zone

The double character start pattern:

- A start character (A, B, or C)
- The Function 1 Symbol Character (FNC1)

Data (including the GS1 Application Identifier represented in character set A, B, or C)

- A symbol check character.
- The stop character.
- Right Quiet Zone.

Two dimensional barcodes - GS1 Data Matrix symbology

GS1 Data Matrix is a standalone, two-dimensional matrix symbology that is made up of square modules arranged within a perimeter finder pattern.

- GS1 Data Matrix has been used in the public domain since 1994.

Data Matrix ISO version ECC 200 is the only version that supports GS1 system data structures, including Function 1 Symbol Character (FNC1). The ECC 200 version of Data Matrix uses Reed Solomon error correction, and this feature helps correct for partially damaged symbols.

the ECC 200 version of Data Matrix is assumed when the symbology is described as GS1 Data Matrix. This version of Data Matrix is similar in stability to ISO versions of current GS1 system symbology's.

GS1 Data Matrix symbols are read by two-dimensional *imaging scanners* or *vision systems*. Most other scanners that are not two-dimensional imagers cannot read GS1 Data Matrix. GS1 Data Matrix symbols are restricted for use with applications that will involve imaging scanners throughout the supply chain.

GS1 Data Matrix features and symbol basics

- GS1 Data Matrix symbol with 20 rows and 20 columns (including the perimeter finder pattern but not including Quiet Zones)

- GS1 Data Matrix solid "L" shaped finder or alignment pattern is one module wide.

- GS1 Data Matrix Quiet Zone is one module wide on all four sides. As with other barcode Quiet Zones, do not print in this area.

- ECC 200 symbols can always be recognised from older versions of Data Matrix because the corner opposite the middle of the finder pattern is a zero module or white in normal print.

- For square GS1 Data Matrix symbols, only an even number of rows and columns exist. Depending on data requirements, symbols can range from 10 row by 10 columns (10 x10) to 144x144 (including finder pattern but not the Quiet Zone).

- ECC 200 (ECC = Error Checking and Correction) that uses Reed-Solomon error correction.

- FNC1 for GS1 system compatibility SHALL be encoded at the beginning of the data string. When a separator character is needed at the end of an element string, either the Function 1 Symbol Character (FNC1) or the control character (ASCII value 29 (decimal), 1D (hexadecimal)) SHALL be used and SHALL be represented in the transmitted message by control character (ASCII value 29 (decimal), 1D (hexadecimal)).

Data characters per symbol (for the maximum symbol size):

- Alphanumeric data: up to 2335 characters.

- Eight-bit byte data: 1556 characters.

- Numeric data: 3116 digits.

GS1 Data Matrix symbology

GS1 Data Matrix symbols shown in the following subsections have been magnified to show detail.

Square and rectangular formats

GS1 Data Matrix may be printed in a square or rectangular format.

- The square format is usually used as it has a larger range of sizes and is the only format available for symbols encoding a large amount of data.

- The largest rectangular symbol can encode 98 digits, while the largest square symbol can encode 3,116 digits.

- An enlarged rectangular symbol and an equivalent square symbol are shown in the figure below.

Data transmission and symbology identifier prefixes

The GS1 system requires the use of symbology identifiers. GS1 Data Matrix uses the symbology identifier of]d2 for GS1 system compliant symbols that have a leading FNC1 character.

Symbology identifier for Data Matrix ECC 200

	Message content	separator
]d2	Standard AI element strings	None

Symbol quality grade

The International Standard ISO/IEC 15415 Information technology - Automatic identification and data capture techniques – Bar code symbol print quality test specification - Two-dimensional symbols methodology SHALL be used for measuring and grading GS1 Data Matrix.

Master Data Sharing With Gs1 Global Data Synchronisation Network

The GS1 Global Data Synchronisation Network, or GDSN®, is another GS1 Communication Standard.

The GDSN is built around the GS1 Global Registry, GDSNcertified Data Pools, the GS1 Data Quality Framework and GS1 Global Product Classification, which, when combined, provide a powerful environment for secure and continuous synchronisation of accurate data.

The GS1 Global Registry is the GDSN's "network facilitator and information directory" that guarantees the uniqueness of the registered items and parties. It provides data pools critical information to establish data synchronisation communications in the network and ensures they are using a standard set of messages, validation rules, and processes.

GDSN-certified Data Pools are electronic catalogues of standardised item data. They serve as a source and/or a recipient of master data. Data Pools can be run by a GS1 Member Organisation or by a solution provider. An up-todate list of all GDSN-certified Data Pools is always available at www.gs1.org/gdsn.

The GS1 Data Quality Framework uses GS1 standards and fits perfectly into GDSN. For suppliers, it enhances internal processes and guarantees the good quality of data that is shared. For retailers, hospitals, pharmacies and other data recipients, it helps ensure that they have the means to receive and use proper information.

To ensure products are classified correctly and uniformly, GDSN uses GS1 Global Product Classification (GPC), a system that gives buyers and sellers a common language for grouping products in the same way, everywhere in the world. This improves the Global Data Synchronisation Network's data accuracy and integrity, speeds up the supply chain's ability to react to consumer needs and contributes to breaking down language barriers. It also facilitates the reporting process across product silos. The foundation of GPC is called a "brick". GPC bricks define categories of similar products. Using the GPC brick as part of GDSN ensures the correct recognition of the product category across the extended supply chain, from seller to buyer.

Transactional Data with GS1 eCom

Every day in companies around the world, hundreds of millions of business transactions take place: orders, order responses, despatches, payments and more. And with increasing regularity, these transactions are being handled electronically.

By using GS1 Identification Keys such as GTIN, GLN and SSCC, GS1 eCom enables the direct integration of data captured during the scanning of products sold in retail, during logistic activities and so forth. It saves users from a costly and time-consuming mapping of proprietary identification schemes – because the same GS1 ID Keys which are used to collect data at the retail point of sales or during logistic activities while despatching and receiving of goods are also used here.

GS1 eCom provides two complementary standards: GS1 EANCOM and GS1 XML. They both allow a direct link between the physical flow of goods or services, and information related to them.

GS1 EANCOM

GS1 EANCOM® is a GS1 eCom Communication standard based on UN/EDIFACT (United Nations Electronic Data Interchange for Administration, Commerce and Transport), which is a set of internationally agreed-upon standards, directories and guidelines for the electronic interchange of data.

The messages available in GS1 EANCOM can be divided into the following categories:

- Master Data Messages

- Business Transactions Messages
- Report and Planning Messages
- Syntax and Service Report Messages
- Security Messages

GS1 XML

XML is an industry acronym for "eXtensible Markup Language," a programming language that was designed for information exchange over the Internet.

GS1 was one of the first standards organisations to publish a global XML-based business standard, and the GS1 XML currently contains more than 60 "document" XML messages, not counting supporting messages from the common library.

GS1 XML messages are also used in the Global Data Synchronisation Network and in event management enabled by RFID via GS1 EPCglobal. GS1 XML is designed in such a way that the messaging is transport agnostic. It is very simple to exchange GS1 XML documents using any technical solution or profile, including Web Services.

GS1 Communication Standards: Visibility Data with EPCIS

Electronic Product Code Information Services, or EPCIS, is another GS1 Communication Standard.

EPCIS answers the questions: What? Where? When? Why?

> **WHAT:**(object identified by a GS1 Key)
>
> **WHERE:**(event location identified by an SGLN)
>
> **WHEN**: (date & time of event)
>
> **WHY:** (business context and object status)

The EPCIS Data Model specifies a standard way to represent visibility information about physical objects, including descriptions of product movements in a supply chain. The main components of the data model include its Electronic Product Code, Event Time, Business Step, Disposition, Read Point, Business Location and Business Transaction. The data model is designed to be extendable by industries and end users without revising the specification itself. For example, EPCIS pilots have included extensions such as Expiration Date, Batch Number and Temperature.

The EPCIS Event Capture Interface specifies a standard way for business applications that generate visibility data to communicate that data to applications that wish to consume it. In many cases, the receiving side of the Event Capture Interface will be a repository, but this is not obligatorily the case.

The EPCIS Query Interface provides a standard way for internal and external systems to request business events from repositories and other sources of EPCIS data using a simple, parameter-driven query language. There are two types of queries – Poll Queries for a synchronous, on-demand response, and Subscription Queries for an asynchronous, scheduled response.

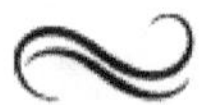

Chapter | 4

Track And Trace System For Supply Chain Visibility

Fundamentals Of The Pharmaceutical Supply Chain

The pharmaceutical supply chain is the means through which prescription medicines are manufactured and delivered to patients. But the supply chain network is actually very complex, requiring a number of steps that must be taken to ensure medications are available and accessible to patients.

> *The pharmaceutical supply chain is complex and pharmaceutical companies must address the most common challenges in order to get patients their needed medications efficiently.*

distributed incorrectly affect both the company's reputation and customer satisfaction, as well

In such a complex process, the stakes are high for pharmaceutical companies. Drugs that are distributed incorrectly affect both the company's reputation and customer satisfaction, as well as potential profit. An ineffective supply chain could also disrupt the healing processes of patients and produce negative effects on public health.

The pharmaceutical supply chain faces its own set of challenges:

- Supply chain visibility
- drug counterfeiting
- Cold-chain shipping
- Raising prescription drug prices which can significantly increase out-of-pocket costs for patients.

How Does the Pharmaceutical Supply Chain Work?

the most basic level, there are five-steps in the pharmaceutical supply chain to ensure that drug inventory is readily available for distribution to providers and patients.

Those five steps are:

1. Pharmaceuticals originate in manufacturing sites.

2. Are transferred to wholesale distributors.

3. Stocked at retail, mail-order, and other types of pharmacies.

4. Subject to price negotiations and processed through quality and utilization management screens by pharmacy benefit management companies.

5. Dispensed by pharmacies; and ultimately delivered to and taken by patients.

How can Serialization Management enhance your Supply Chain?

One of the constant battles the pharmaceutical industry has to face, is to prevent counterfeit and falsified drugs from entering the market and putting the public's health at risk.

The fraudulent products and drugs may be manufactured in multiple locations (fillers in one location, packaging in another, etc). It makes identifying them difficult to track and trace in order for them to be removed from the supply chain. With serialization of these goods, a unique serial number is assigned to each saleable unit per product. It makes having the necessary information about the origin, batch number and expiration date of the product easy to identify throughout the entire supply chain — from production till it reaches the patient.

A robust serialization management strategy can benefit not just the manufacturer, but the entire supply chain. With serialization of products, there's trust, responsibility, transparency and ownership between all the members (manufacturers, stakeholders and customers) in the supply chain.

Serialization allows supply chains to become more efficient as it makes tracking and tracing products easier as well as recalling and returns of products quicker and simpler. This also helps businesses plan better and reduce overhead costs. They can prevent stock piling of excess products as serialization helps in understanding which products are in demand, how much production is needed and how much cost to allocate for manufacturing.

Organizations can prevent unforeseen and costly supply-chain disruptions and vulnerabilities that lead to recalls by strengthening their risk management. Businesses should factor in current events (political and economic) to forecast their impact on manufacturing, production and operations. Businesses should also be able to identify and document potential risk in the future, design and use methodology that has provided high value solutions. This may allow them to be in a position to replace products speedily for better customer service. In this manner companies can trace counterfeit products down to the unit level and also speedily act upon product shortages.

Supply chains may experience blockages at times owing to changing global regulations and restrictions. The governing authorities per country may have specific requirements and it crucial for businesses to be aware of these to prevent delays. Serialization can help in being compliant and meet the required regulations.

How To Drive Successful Serialization In The Supply Chain?

The pharmaceutical industry has been able to prevent excess flooding of counterfeit and harmful products in the supply chain by ensuring compliance measures for serialization and traceability processes are followed. By implementing unique identifiers (such as unique serial numbers) for products and adhering to rules set by regulatory bodies, the industry has been able to adopt serialization for their products.

What more can be done in the industry to improve the processes for serializing products and to build a more efficient supply chain?

1. Strengthen data exchange networks

2. Incorporate sustainable solutions

Strengthening Data Exchange Networks

- Strengthen and support data exchange between various networks which can improve implementation and help them have access to accurate insights throughout the supply chain.

- serialization can help make distribution of products safer and quicker so it reaches patients in a timely manner. With accurate data platforms and the right analytical tools,

- Markets in the industry seem to be heavily stressing on exchange of serialization data between different markets so it can make traceability of a product easier around the world.

- As one of the most recent trends being adopted within the pharma industry has been investing in blockchain technology, this has further allowed networks and trading partners to have efficient data exchange take place between them.

Incorporating Sustainable Serialization Solutions

- The serialization programs businesses adopt should look at meeting all the requirements and balance all the day to day operations.

- Organization events will need to factor in looking at serialization and traceability requirements in new or existing markets, network changes and transfers, mergers and acquisitions, new business opportunities and relationships that include marketing, distribution and co-licensing as well as factoring in recalls, audits, investigations and complaints.

Businesses should look at developing strategies that include sustainable solutions and to begin with can factor in:

- **Sustainable digitization for packaging** – this can help with anti-counterfeiting of products through serialized labels, etc.

- Create sustainable strategies for increased and cost-effective ROI – this should include market changes for changing and country specific serialization regulations, supply chain interconnectivity and all future technologies in the supply chain such as the use of *AI* and as mentioned earlier, *Blockchain.*

Steps to help you improve transparency in your supply chain

Here are basic steps you can implement to start you off on your journey.

1. **Risk assessment and Setting an Outcome:**

There are several ways in which you can complete a risk assessment. Often companies will create a plan detailing internal processes and participants and external collaborators and contributors. This is known as a materiality assessment. This can be done by looking at looming hazards due to the passing of new laws and policies, disturbances in the economy, and past problems with suppliers.

2. **Envision the supply chain:**

Once you have pinpointed the problems and itemized them, try to imagine what your ideal supply chain looks like. It will help you better understand the passage of goods, outline the vendors and their intersection of procedures, and reveal any gaps of knowledge. This information should be in line with your chosen outcome.

3. **Gather information you can act on:**

Once you have outlined your supply chain, gather data on procedures and fulfillments that gives you an insight into possible risks, openings for improvement, and knowledge gaps. You may need to track and trace individual elements, groups, or shipments travelling through your supply train to verify chain of custody and origin point.

As you confirm your chain of custody, you will have to solidify your company procedures and ensure that they are being followed at every step – this can cover anything from the labour policies of vendors to environmental regulations. You can get this directly from your vendors, but of late with the increase in regulations, companies may ask external contractors to implement the former's own policies and practices.

4. **Participation:**

Once you have the relevant information, you can now choose how to modulate participation in your supply chain. This will usually entail a plan of action considering crucial KPIs. Companies should be looking to affect targeted problems like clarifying source points, ensuring compliance with labour laws and regulations, and any adverse environmental impact by vendors. You may have to collaborate with outside parties to fill any knowledge gaps that cannot be filled internally.

5. **Reporting:**

The final step is to select the depth of reporting your company is willing to do. This involves sharing information with shareholders, ensuring fulfillment of governmental compliance, and verification of the reports. The companies have various options at this stage, from sharing company policy to releasing a map of the entire supply chain.

Those are five basic steps you can implement to improve traceability in your supply chain. Do keep in mind that supply chains are ever-changing and reacting, whether it be to changes in the economy of new government regulations. This process to improve traceability should be ongoing and frequently reviewed. While the implementation of technology such as Blockchain can help in this matter, the final answer will entail the right balance of manpower, data, and technology which supports your desired outcome.

Growing the Pharmaceutical Supply Chain

Blockchain Technology is able to provide businesses a secure and quick transaction across the globe. In the pharmaceutical industry, it is also being used for clinical trials, to track and trace drugs that are manufactured or shipped and for all aspects of maintaining essential records (identity, transactions, contracts, etc).

The industry can really leverage this technology by applying it within supply chains. It can help create a trail that's auditable and can benefit businesses greatly by establishing drug provenance across the supply chain with just one software. This can allow manufacturers and their consumers to easily access, verify the quality of the drugs as well as the origins of it. As everyone within the supply chain ecosystem has access to all the data real time and there's transparency at every stage of the supply chain journey, it can prevent counterfeiting, tampering, diversions and make tracking-and-tracing quicker. Any changes to the records are displayed for all to see and this makes product recalls simpler for businesses who can identify and pull out the faulty production batches.

supply chain analytics and visibility software
Economical and integrated end-to-end supply chain visibility, with AI monitored serialization at item, box and pallet level.

An Advanced Digital Supply Chain Analytics Platform
- Scalable
- Fully integrated
- Comprehensive
- Extensible

Problems That Are Solved Out-Of-The-Box
- Real-time visibility all the way to the consumers with geo-location.
- Instant verification and validation of the origin to prevent leaks.
- Distribution terms on big retailers and online sellers are enforceable
- Retailers will avoid grey distributors as Brands can trace the PoS.

- Protection from legal liability caused by illegal shipment or smuggling by others.

- Instant activation of recall with complete visibility.

- Centralized information about the current and dead stock in every warehouse and distribution center.

- Real-time and accurate product performance analytics with geo-location

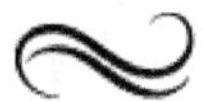

Chapter | 5

Data Notifications & Management

Overview

Many serialization regulations require that pharmaceutical entities track each saleable unit throughout the supply chain. Most regulations require a serial number to be unique across a product. Some regulations require a serial number to be unique across all of the products manufactured by a company.

With at least 75 percent of the global drug supply requiring track and trace regulation by early 2019, companies are focused on addressing the complexities of serialization.

One major complexity is the maintenance and exchange of information about each product, source, and destination. Such information—known as master data—is integral to both the packaging and labelling process and the data exchange requirements involved with serialization.

Understanding the impact of master data on compliance will help you determine how to plan your serialization strategy.

Every serial number must be accompanied by master data as it journeys through the supply chain. Master Data Management.

Defining Master Data

Master data functions as a single source of truth to build a reliable system of record—no matter where the data is encountered in the supply chain. Master data defines the contextual attributes of a data object at a foundational level by describing elements such as product name, a price list, or a partner shipping address. It can be helpful to think of master data as the nouns in business data: company location, unit of measure, dosage form, contact email, or government drug code.

Master data interacts with transactional data.

Think of transactional data as the set of verbs in business data: sale, shipment, or decommissioning of a product.

Pairing master and transactional data streamline the number of data elements sent to disparate compliance systems throughout the supply chain.

Master data creation

- Master data is created only once, in one place, and then reused repeatedly and stored in many systems, such as an ERP or government repository.
- It is constantly being added, removed, or edited within a dataset.

- Adding a new site or partner location contact requires data such as GLN or other identifiers, while a new product may require manufacturer name and packaging code type.

- Different companies may refer to products or partners in different ways, so efforts to synchronize such information must be made. Since it lives in multiple places, master data is at risk of becoming inaccurate, redundant, or stale if vigilance and best practices are not employed.

Key Types Of Master Data

Company Master Data Contains a record for each of your company's locations, including address and company identifiers such as GLN and DUNS number, country code, business logo, and business type.

Partner Master Data identifies your partners and their locations using attributes describing addresses, contact information, and global identifiers, such as DEA, HIN, DUNS, or State License.

Product Master Data is a list of all your products and their descriptive information. When adding a new product, you might need to include elements such as target market code, product name and description, currency code, unit price, strength, GTIN, or aggregation requirements.

The Importance Of Master Data For Serialization

In serialization, you are applying serial numbers to a given product, case, or other packaging unit, so you need a defined set of attributes that a track and trace system can use to manage data.

Ultimately, master data is referenced during data exchange between numerous internal and external interfaces and is used to ensure that core information gets to the right place and is aligned with the right serial number.

When companies begin thinking about serialization, they often focus at first on just the serial number, and then on transactional data—with the foundational aspects of master data often getting overlooked.

An inherent part of compliance reporting, your master data must be well-defined and clearly managed. If you focus just on the packaging line and how to get a serial number on a package, then you are likely to run into challenges later because you have not accounted for master data usage throughout the entire serialization process.

What is master data management?

Master data management concern the technology and processes used for the ongoing maintenance of master data. To protect the health of your master data.

Key objective

Accuracy: Give operators the change to enter data correctly.

Availability: Optimize search features and minimize interruptions.

Quality: Minimize errors and protect your brand.

Integrity: Protect your systems and your patients.

The Risks: The Impact Of Master Data Errors

Having incorrect or incomplete master data can result in compliance reporting errors throughout all segments of the supply chain.

In a typical CMO integration, for example, serial number structure and forms are validated against the CMO partner master data and the product master data attributes that an authorised CMO will produce. The validation and acceptance of serial numbers relies on the serial number flow.

This flow can be disrupted, and cause system errors, when a piece of master data is incorrect.

Incomplete or erroneous master data may result in additional significant risks, including:

- Patient safety data.
- Compliance costs for corrections and development of more efficient processes.
- Risk to the rest of supply chain.
- Trade partner satisfaction.
- Heavy fines.
- Legal exposure.
- Risk to company image and investor perception.

Master Data Exchange For Serialization And Track And Trace

Processes and techniques regarding the identification of static data and processes to keep the data up to date. Emphasizes implementation of one source for master data and referencing the data using standardized identifiers.

Application for serialisation

- Master Data Exchange

- Serial Number Manager

- Serial Number Exchange

- Serialized Operations Manager

Master Data Exchange application provides a repository to manage the master data required for serialization, track and trace, and compliance requirements. Although many companies have invested in master data management systems, these systems typically do not contain all of the master data elements requirements for compliance. They are also not easily accessible to third party applications.

With Master Data Exchange you can:

- Maintain master data for company and locations, trade partners, and products.

- Consolidate master data required for serialization, track and trace, and compliance into a single repository.

- Enrich transactions with master data so that master data does not need to be included in every transaction.

- Trigger business logic and workflow based on data captured in master data, such as product target market.

- Integrate to the master data system of record to ensure data is continuously kept up to date.

- Manually populate master data through CSV or XML files and user interface data entry.

Serial Number Manager

- Serial Number Manager application provides serial number generation functionality in compliance with industry standards and regulations.

- Serial numbers are generated against user-defined serial number templates that control the serial number format, length, and algorithm by product and packaging level.

- Serial number templates also define the minimum and maximum serial number inventories by product so that serial numbers are always available for packaging runs.

With Serial Number Manager you can:

- Define the serial number generation rules needed to meet your compliance and business requirements.

- Create serial number templates for your products at the item, case, pallet, and other packaging levels required for a market Support packaging code types including GTIN-14, SSCC, NTIN, and China Res Codes.

- Encode serial numbers using AI (01)+AI(21), AI(00), and CN-EDMC encoding types

- Create serial numbers using sequential list, sequential range, and randomized generation algorithms

- Ensure serial numbers are always available by specifying a minimum threshold for each product

- Auto-replenish serial numbers from external serial number management systems

- Track number of remaining serial numbers available in the serial number pool

- Allow contract packagers or third-party label providers to create serial numbers on your behalf

Serial Number Exchange

- Serial Number Exchange provides functionality governing the allocation of serial numbers to packaging lines and contract partners.

- Serial Number Exchange manages the request of serial numbers from line management systems and provides the response as well as the processing of commissioning and aggregation information.

- Serial Number Exchange includes configurable business logic that controls from what products and locations serial numbers can be requested. Serial Number Exchange also includes business logic that verifies commission and aggregation information received from the packaging line to detect abnormalities and errors.

With Serial Number Exchange you can:

- Request, commission, aggregate, disaggregate, and repackage serial numbers

- Verify serial numbers to ensure they are commissioned to the correct product and allocated to the site performing the commissioning

- Create production orders

- Report an end of batch

- Transfer serial numbers between sites

- Update serial number status when destroying, decommissioning, or deactivating serial numbers

- Encode serial numbers in order to transfer them to third-party printers

- Manage exceptions by site

Serialized Operations Manager

Serialized Operations Manager (SOM) application provides an EPCIS repository to manage events associated with serialization data. In addition, Serialized Operations Manager enables supply chain and distribution processes so that serialization does not need to be embedded into ERP and WMS systems.

With Serialized Operations Manager you can:

- Insulate your ERP and WMS from needing knowledge of serialization data

- Track and manage serialized product post packaging

- Manage aggregation and disaggregation processes

- Monitor the current state and history of serialized inventory

- Execute supply chain transactions such as receipts, transfers, and shipments of serialized product

- Execute business logic based on EPCIS event data and master data

- Integrate an edge device layer to enable serialization on the warehouse floor

Serialization Profile

The serialization profile is the blue print of the range definition and defines how serial numbers are composed

The profile contains the following attributes

Profile key: This is the external identifier of the serialization profile.

Serial Number Length: Most legislations foresee a serial number length of maximum 20 digits.

Serial Number Type:.

Defines the allowed character set for the generation of serial numbers. Following types are supported.

Numeric: Allows numbers from 0-9.

- Alphanumeric (capital letters): Allows numbers from 0-9 and the 26 capital characters from the Latin alphabet (A-Z). Further characters (for example, special Characters, punctuation marks, umlaut, and so on) are not supported.

- Alphanumeric (case sensitive): Allows numbers from 0-9 and the 52 characters from the Latin alphabet (a-z and A-Z). Further characters (for example, special Characters, punctuation marks, umlaut, and so on) are not supported.

- Alphanumeric (case sensitive) with exclusion list: Allows numbers from 0-9 and the 52 characters from the Latin alphabet (a-z and A-Z). Further characters (for example, special Characters, punctuation marks, umlaut, and so on) are not supported.

Serial Number Randomization Mode: Defines how the randomization of serial numbers is done. Following randomization modes are supported:

- Non-randomized

- Randomized 1:100

- Randomized 1:1000

- Randomized 1:10000

- Combined Sequential number. + 3 Digit Randomized

- Combined Sequential number. + 4 Digit Randomized

- Manual Randomization

- External Randomization

Uniqueness Scope: The serial number uniqueness scope defines how unique a serial number is. The following uniqueness scopes are supported.

- By Trade item
- By country portfolio
- Globally

Serial Number

Use

Ranges of type List managed and Range and list managed can handle serial numbers. Every serial number created is a unique instance and can be followed individually throughout its life cycle. The serial number status denotes the current phase of the serial number in its life cycle.

Given below are the most important attributes of a Serial Number:

Range Definition Name and Version

- **Serial Number GTIN:** Trade item for which the serial number has been requested.

- **GCP**: Global Company Prefix for which the serial number has been requested.

- **System:** This denotes the system that requested the serial number. A serial number in status created has no system assigned. Only after the serial number has been requested by and sent to an own system (status assigned / sent) the system is added to the serial number.

- **Serial Number Status:** The serial number supports following status values:

- 0 – Created

- 1 – Assigned/Send

- 2 – Commissioned

- 3 – Reported Lost

- **Generated on: Dat**e and time when the serial number was generated

- **Sent on:** Date and time when the serial number was sent to a consumer via a serial number list request.

- **Updated on:** Date and time when the last update was made to the serial number

Activities

You can perform the following actions in the results pane:

- Create a Serial Number List Request

- Change the status of a serial number: Individual serial numbers can be declared as lost. Select one or more lines in the result list and execute action change status Report as lost.

- View related serial number

- View related serial number

- Generation of Serial Numbers

Creation of Serial Numbers

Process

- Once the serial number is generated, it is in the *created status*. The generation time reflects the date and time of the number generation. GTIN, GCP, and System are not populated after generation of the number as the serial number is not dedicated for a GTIN or GCP yet.

- After the system requests the serial number, the status of the number is assigned/send.

- During commissioning, the system determines if the serial number was requested by the same business partner when compared to the one commissioning the serial number. Only if this check succeeds, the SGTIN can be commissioned using the serial number. In this case, the status of the serial number is updated to commissioned and the update time stamp reflects the date and time of the commissioning. The status commissioned is one of two final status values.

Serial Number Generation and Randomization

Randomize unique serial numbers based on two algorithms with different flavours.

Process
Serial Number Generation

Serial numbers are always pre-generated to allow fast responding serial number requests. The two most important parameters to trigger number generation are threshold and lot size.

- The threshold defines the quantity of serial numbers that is always available for requests. When the threshold is reached by a request, the system triggers the serial number generation automatically.

- The lot size defines the quantity of serial numbers that is generated in one generation run.

Randomization Mode

Non-randomized: no randomization; only sequential number management.

Randomized 1:100: For example, if the range carries 10000 numbers, you can pick only 100 numbers from this range.

Randomized 1:1000: For example, if the range carries 10000 numbers, only 10 numbers can be picked from this range.

Randomized 1:10000: For example, if the range carries 10000 numbers, only 1 number can be picked from this range.

Chapter | 6

Serialization And Traceability Requirements Of Regulatory Legislations.

Introduction

The national regulations on the serialization and aggregation of drugs are possibly the most important criteria in the global marketing of pharmaceuticals and other related healthcare solutions. Optimum implementation requires *complete and up-to-the-minute knowledge of the relevant obligations* for pharma serialization and aggregation.

Supply chains for pharmaceutical manufacturing production are becoming increasingly complex. Medications, from source to shelf, now involve numerous networks and cross the borders of many different countries around the globe. Serialisation requirements in the pharmaceutical industry have become an important part of this complex production process.

> *According to W.H.O*
>
> ***"Counterfeit medications yield over $10 billion annually and result in thousands of deaths".***
>
> ***"1 in 10 medications in developing countries have been found to be counterfeit"***

> *"Serialisation means the application of a unique random serial number on each saleable unit of pharmaceutical product, which can be traced back to the original source of supply".*

Serialisation Requirements (Globally)

- Most countries have increased labelling regulation requirements (GMP requirements for packaging and labelling) to include the concept of serialisation. Countries like the European union, China and South Korea and the U.S. have already regulated the concept of serialisation.

- Serialisation has been mandated in approximately 80% of countries across the globe, to minimise the risks of fraudulent drugs entering the market.

> *"If you have not yet implemented serialisation of your secondary packaging, you will be ineligible to supply your pharmaceutical products to the countries those who have implemented serialisation regulations."*

US Drug Supply Chain Security Act (DSCSA)

- The Drug Quality and Security Act (DQSA), was enacted by Congress on November 27, 2013.

- Title II of DQSA, the Drug Supply Chain Security Act (DSCSA), outlines steps to build an electronic, interoperable system to identify and trace certain prescription drugs as they are distributed in the United States.

- This will enhance FDA's ability to help protect consumers from exposure to drugs that may be counterfeit, stolen, contaminated, or otherwise harmful.

- The system will also improve detection and removal of potentially dangerous drugs from the drug supply chain to protect U.S. consumers.

Regulation agencies

1. U.S. Department of Health and Human Services (HHS): also known as the Health Department, is a cabinet-level executive branch department of the U.S. federal government with the goal of protecting the health of all Americans and providing essential human services. Its motto is "Improving the health, safety, and well-being of America".

2. Food and Drug Administration (US FDA): The Food and Drug Administration is responsible for protecting the public health by ensuring the safety, efficacy, and security of human and veterinary drugs, biological products, and medical devices; and by ensuring the safety of our nation's food supply, cosmetics, and products that emit radiation.

Regulation Name: The Drug Supply Chain Security Act (DSCSA), which is Title II of the Drug Quality and Security Act (DQSA)

Title II: Drug Supply Chain Security Act (DSCSA)

Title II of the act, the Drug Supply Chain Security Act (DSCSA), established requirements to facilitate the tracing of prescription drug products through the pharmaceutical supply distribution chain.

Under DSCSA, the Secretary is required to establish standards for the exchange of transaction documentation, including transaction information, transaction history, and transaction statements. The Secretary must also establish processes to provide waivers of requirements, including for undue economic hardship or emergency medical reasons provide exceptions to requirements relating to product identifiers if a product is packaged without sufficient space to bear the information; and determine other products or transactions that should be exempt from the requirements of the act.

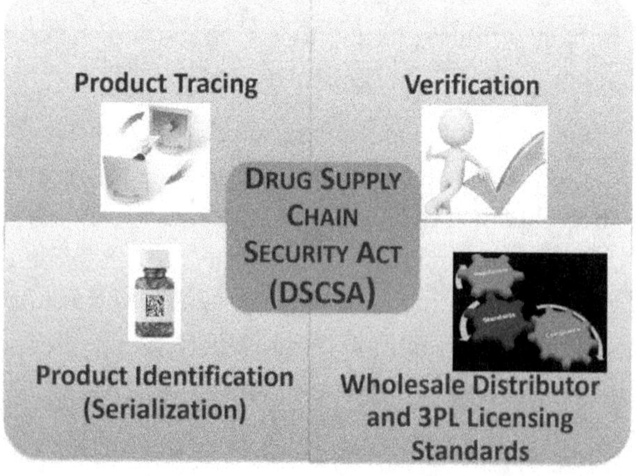

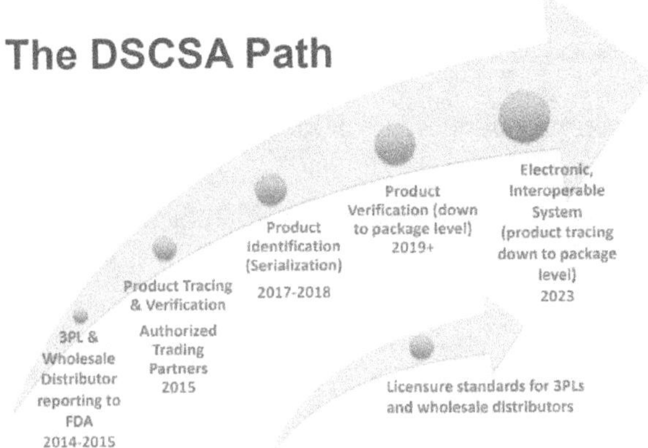

Requirements

The act established requirements for drug manufacturers, wholesalers, dispensers, and repackagers:

Summary of Requirements and Affected Parties

Requirement	Manufacturer	Repackager	Wholesaler	Dispenser
Provide prior transaction information at each transfer of ownership	Yes	Yes	Yes	Yes
Provide transaction documentation the event of a recall or for the purpose of investigating a suspect product or an illegitimate product	Yes	Yes	Yes	Yes
Ensure that all of one's trading partners are authorized	Yes	Yes	Yes	Yes
Affix or imprint a product identifier on each package and homogenous case	Yes	Yes	No	No
Implement systems to investigate suspect products and handle illegitimate products	Yes	Yes	Yes	Yes

Verify returned products before further distribution	Yes	Yes	Yes	No

The act pre-empts state and local requirements related to tracing drugs through the distribution system, and licensure of wholesale distributors and third-party logistics providers.

The DSCSA Timeline:

Deadline	Impacted	Requirements
January, 1st 2015	Manufacturers	Lot number printed on packaging of Rx drugs
November, 27th 2017	Manufacturers	GTIN + serial number + lot number + expiry date in human-readable format and GS1 data matrix
November, 27th 2018	Repackagers	Serialization for repackaged medicines
November, 27th 2019	Wholesalers	Authentication & verification
November, 27th 2020	Dispensers	Authentication & verification
November, 27th 2023	Whole pharma supply chain	Complete unit level traceability including aggregation throughout the whole supply chain

DCSCA: Key Provisions and Compliance Requirements

- Product identification.
- Product tracing.
- Product verification.
- Detection and response – suspect and illegitimate.
- Notification.

- Wholesaler licensing.

- Third-party logistics provider licensing.

- T3
  - ✓ Transaction Information
  - ✓ Transaction Statement
  - ✓ Transaction History

Track & Receive Lot Level Compliance Data: Stakeholders must be able to receive the lot-level Transaction History (TH), Transaction Information (TI), and Transaction Statement (TS) compliance documentation for every product they purchase. "T3"

Verify "T3"Compliance Data: Stakeholders verify the "T3" Compliance Data against the product that was shipped to them by their suppliers, and must quarantine any product they determine to be suspect or questionable.

Store "T3"Compliance Data: Stakeholders must store the compliance information associated with every shipment they receive for a period of at least 6 years from the date of shipment receipt.

2D Bar Code and Requirements

Product Identifier: A GS-1-compliant standardized graphic that includes, in both human-readable form and on a machine-readable data carrier:

- The standardized numerical identifier,

- Lot number

- Expiration date of the product.

Standardized Numerical Identifier (SNI): A set of numbers or characters used to uniquely identify each package or homogenous case that is composed of the National Drug Code that corresponds to the specific product (including the particular package configuration) combined with a unique alphanumeric serial number of up to 20 characters.

Package: The smallest individual saleable unit of product for distribution by a Manufacturer or Repackager that is intended by the Manufacturer for ultimate sale to the Dispenser of such product.

(01)00300011234013	GTIN
(21) 123456789012	Serial Number
(17) 01 2023	Expiry date
(10) A123456X	Batch number

For illustration purpose only

Bar Code Symbology: ECC-200 GS1 Data Matrix.

Bar Code Data Structure – Data Matrix Code.

Data to be encoded in the Data Matrix code:

- Product Identification Number (GTIN) – AI(01)
- Serial Number – AI(21)
- Expiration Date – AI(17)
- Lot Number – AI(10)

Data Structure Analysis shall be in accordance with the table below:

Note the FNC1 at the beginning of the string and between the Serial Number and Expiration Date to identify the end of the variable length field (i.e., Serial Number) and the beginning of the fixed length field (i.e., Expiration Date). Although Lot Number is also a variable length field, a FNC1 is not required as it is at the end of the string.

Embedded Data	Description	Value
<232>	FNC 1	<FNC 1>
01	GTIN	(01)
00300011234013	GTIN	00300011234013
21	Serial Number	(21)
123456789012	Serial Number	123456789012
<232>	FNC 1	<FNC 1>
17	Expiration Date (YYMMDD)	(17)
230131	Expiration Date (YYMMDD)	230131
10	Batch Number	(10)
A123456X	Batch Number	A123456X

Bar Code Size: a 26x26 symbol size it may be varied.

Bar Code Quiet Zone: For 2D codes it is a minimum of 3 times the X dimension or 0.1 inch recommended.

Bar Code Quality: The print quality grade shall be at least 1.5 (adequate) in accordance with ISO/IEC 15415:2011.

NEW Returns Requirements

- Distributors must associate the original Transaction Information, Transaction History and Transactional Statement with a saleable return.

- Verify that the product identifier affixed to the product corresponds with the data the manufacturer assigned.

  ✓ Manufacturers can send serialized data for their shipments to their trading partners to be used for verification of future saleable returns.

--OR--

  ✓ Manufacturers can make serial data available for query using a Verification Router Service requesting data for the distributors.

Returns Verification

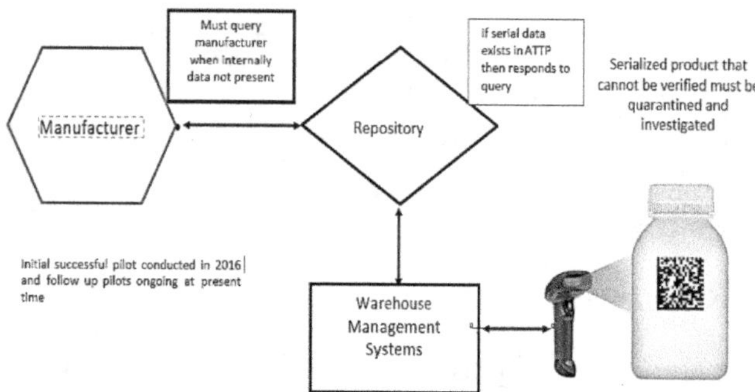

2023 Requirements of DSCSA

The pharmaceutical industry of America completed the serialization of all drugs project in 2017-2018. The next most aggressive challenge is to ensure that serialized drugs are traceable within the supply chain. Serialized drugs need to be aggregated to make sure that the drugs are traceable in the supply chain. In addition, pharmaceutical manufacturers are required to install a VRS (Verification Router Services) system.

Aggregation For Full Compliance With DSCSA.

Drugs on the US market and transport units that integrate these drugs (container case, bundle, pallet) have been serialized. But the DSCSA wants hierarchical aggregation of transport units. What does this mean?

In short, aggregation in the pharmaceutical industry is defined as the virtual connection of serialized transport units and serialized drugs within them. The most common method for this virtual connection is to create a hierarchical data with a parent-child relationship. When this data is associated with the serialized transport unit, the aggregation is complete.

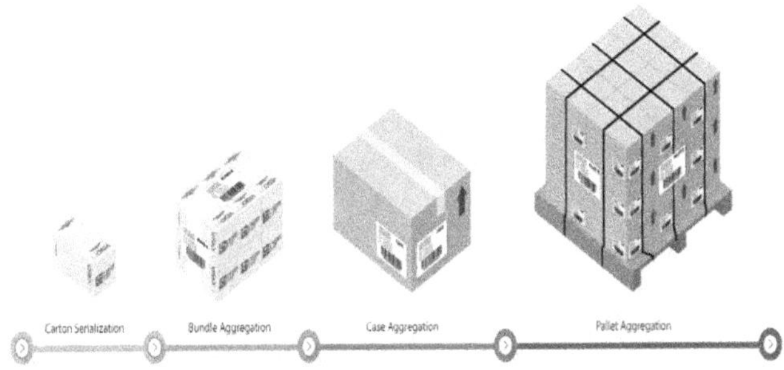

Serialization - Challenges and Risk

- Manufacturers are already applying 2D barcodes on Product

- Electronic Format – Compliance

- Supply chain organizations and 2023

- FDA Enforcement Discretion

European Union Falsified Medicine Directive (2011/62/Eu)

Overview:

- *9 February, 2019* marked as delegated Regulation's compliance date.

- The impacted all *Rx Medicines* with marketing authorization's Requiring them to carry:

  ✓ *Tamper evidence* closures to ensure product integrity.

  ✓ *Unique identifier* to allow each individual barcode to be verified.

  ✓ Authenticity of Unique identifier is checked Using a network of ***medicine verification systems.***

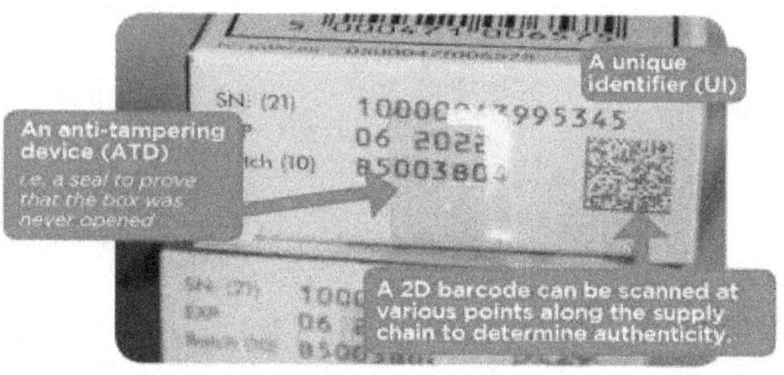

Safety features	
Unique identifiers	Anti-Tamper Devices
2D Data Matrix	Security seal
ECC-200 (FNC1)	HMG carton, VOID Stickers etc.

What is EU FMD Mandate?

On February 9, 2016, the Delegated Act on safety features detailing implementation requirements for the EU Falsified Medicines Directive was published in the Official Journal of the European Union. With this publication, the regulations for coding, serialization, compliance reporting and verification as described in the Delegated Act now become binding on the EU member states

Implementation timelines for the EU regulatory requirements, based on the publication date, are as follows:

February 9, 2019 – EU Member States (excluding Italy, Greece) EEA members (Norway, Iceland, Liechtenstein) Switzerland

February 9, 2025 – Italy, Greece.

Unique Identifier requirements: DATA-Matrix Code, developed to ISO-standards, including Product code, unique serial number, Expiry date, Batch number, National health number (Wherever necessary)

Falsified medicines: overview

Falsified medicines do not pass through the usual evaluation of quality, safety and efficacy that is required for the EU authorisation procedure. Because of this, they can be a **health threat**.

Until recently, the most frequently falsified medicines in wealthy countries were expensive **'lifestyle' medicines**, such as hormones, steroids and antihistamines. In developing countries, they have included medicines used to treat **life-threatening conditions** such as malaria, tuberculosis and HIV / AIDS.

The phenomenon of <u>falsified medicines</u> is **on the increase**, with more and more medicines now being falsified. These include expensive medicines, such as anticancer medicines, and medicines in high demand, such as antivirals.

Falsified vs. counterfeit medicines

Falsified medicines are not the same as counterfeit medicines:

- <u>Falsified medicines</u> are fake medicines that are designed to mimic real medicines.

- <u>Counterfeit medicines</u> are medicines that do not comply with intellectual-property rights or that infringe trademark law.

Legal framework

In July 2011, the EU strengthened the protection of patients and consumers by adopting a new DIRECTIVE 2011/62/EU on falsified medicines for human use.

The Directive came into force on 21 July 2011. Member States had to start applying its measures in January 2013.

his Directive aims to prevent falsified medicines entering the legal supply chain and reaching patients.

Four main pillars:

1. **Safety features of medicines**

- unique identifier (a 2-dimension barcode) and an anti-tampering device, in accordance with <u>Commission Delegated Regulation (EU) 2016/161</u>.

- Manufacturers will upload the information contained in the unique identifier for each individual medicine to a central EU repository.

- The repository is part of an end-to-end medicines verification system introduced by the Regulation.

- Depending on the source of the medicine, wholesalers will also need to scan medicines at different points in the supply chain to verify their authenticity.

- These safety features will guarantee medicine authenticity for the benefit of patients and businesses.

  1. **Supply chain and** good distribution practice

  2. Active substances **and** excipients

  3. **Internet sales**

- The Directive has introduced an obligatory logo that will appear on the websites of legally operating online pharmacies and approved retailers in the EU.

- The logo will allow patients and consumers to identify authorised online pharmacies and approved retailers providing authentic, authorised medicines. Clicking on the logo will link to the national regulatory authority websites, where all legally operating online pharmacies and approved retailers in their respective countries will be listed.

European Pack Coding Guidelines

The European Medicinal Pack Coding Specification

- **Recommendation of GS1 Standard / 2D Data** Matrix

- the EFPIA board recommended the adoption of a unique standard for the coding of pharmaceutical product across Europe based on the *Data Matrix*

ECC-200 to be introduced on all secondary packaging of prescription products sold in Europe.

- The pack/item code will be accompanied by human readable text. The human readable text will be in a font and size that are in accordance with country specific requirements or GS1 recommendations depending on local requirement.

Accommodation of National Numbers

- National numbers may be required within the code in specific situations. The GS1 General Specifications have been extended to accommodate the inclusion of national product identifiers. This capability is provided by the use of NHRN (National Health Reimbursement Numbers) which can be added to the data content of the code using the appropriate Application Identifiers (AI's).

Content of the 2D Code

- The recommendation for coding of pharmaceutical products is to encode in a Data Matrix code a minimum of four items of data.

  1. the product code,

  2. the serial number,

  3. the expiry date and

  4. the lot number (batch code).

Note: Some markets may require the addition of a national number to the code.

The Product Code

The preferred (by manufacturers) implementation for the product Code is to use the GS1 GTIN (Global Trade Item

Number) however the European Hub and thus EMVS supports both ***GTIN/NTIN*** and ***PPN*** coding schemes.

The four critical aspects for the GTIN element are:

1. It must be preceded by the application identifier 01.

2. It must have a code length of 14 digits.

3. It must use a GS1 standard checksum in the 14th digit.

4. It must adhere to the GS1 use for the first digit:

   a. For a sales unit a 0 is required.

   b. For identification of higher package levels, the range is 1-8. (the value 9 has a special defined meaning – ref GS1 specifications.)

Examples of NTINs in use in Europe and formation rules:

Market	NTIN formation rules
Austria	908888 + PZN + check digit
France	3400 + CIP/ACL Code + check digit
Germany	4150 + 8-digit PZN + check digit
Spain	847000 + Codigo Nacional
Sweden, Finland, Denmark, Iceland, Norway	704626 + Nordic Drug Code issued by Nordic Number office + check digit
Switzerland	7680 + Code assigned by Swiss medic (consists of 5 digits Product License number + 3 digits Pack Size indicator) + check digit

The Serial Number

- The serial number is preceded by the *AI 21* and adheres to the GS1 specification where this field is a variable length (up to 20) alphanumeric field followed by a Group Separator (GS) character (to delimit it from the next field unless it is the last field).

- The serial number will be unique per product code.

Randomisation

- The probability that a valid serial number can be guessed should be less than 1 in 10,000 (i.e. < 0.0001).

- Serial IDs shall not be reused within the longer of a) Exp Date +1 year or b) five years.

The Expiry Date

- This field will conform to GS1 standards and is preceded with the AI 17. It is a fixed 6-digit field with the digits representing YYMMDD.

The Lot Number (Batch Code)

- The lot number (batch code) conforms to GS1 standards and is preceded with the AI of 10 and is a variable length field of up to 20 alphanumeric digits followed by a Group Separator (GS) character (to delimit it from the next field unless it is the last field)

The National Healthcare Reimbursement Number (NHRN)

The NHRN is usually assigned by a national authority to healthcare brand owners for specific trade items and shall only be used for compliance to regulatory requirements where the GTIN alone in a bar code symbol will not meet the requirements. Use of NHRN on the item is controlled by and subject to the rules and regulations of national/regional agencies.

The National Healthcare Reimbursement Number		
Application Identifier	NHRN Length	Organization
710	X1 Variable length X20	Germany (IFA)
711	X1 Variable length X20	France (CIP)
712	X1 Variable length X20	Spain
713	X1 Variable length X20	Brazil (Anvisa)
714	X1 Variable length X20	Portugal

Additional NHRN AI's can be requested through the GS1 GSMP.

Where the NHRN is required, the data set will need to include more than four elements;

1. The GTIN (which will be provided by the manufacturing organisation)

2. The Expiry Date

3. The Lot Number

4. The Serial ID and

5. The NHRN.

Pack Code Attributes

Data Element Description	Application Identifier	Example Data
Product Code	01	05060141900015
Expiry Date	17	190200
Batch Number/Lot Code	10	ABC123992

| Serial Number | 21 | 28574abczz3456 |
| NHRN | 710 | 45678912 |

The data encoded into the Data Matrix code for this example would be:

]d20105060141900015171902001OABC1239922128574abczz345671045678912

Pack Code Size

- Small module sizes should be avoided where possible to increase the readability of the code and avoid the need to use specialised code marking equipment.

Pack Code Quality

The quality of the Data Matrix code printing applied to the pack should be 1.5 (C) or better in accordance with ISO/TEC 15415:2011, and printed using ECC200 error correction and will utilise ASCII encoding according to ISO 16022. The use of ASCII encoding is to ensure maximal interoperability with code reading devices likely to be used in the field.

Human Readable Representation

Human Readable Representation	
Field Name	Preferred Prefix
Product Code	PC
Expiry date	EXP
Batch Number/Lot Code	Lot
Serial Number	SN
NHRN	NN

Country specific guidelines
Country: Austria

Product Code: NTIN for single market packs, GTIN for packs shared with other markets	**Sample illustration purpose**
Prefix Prompts: PC: SN: Verwendbar bis: Ch.-B:	PC: 01234567890123 SN: XXX000000XXX Verwendbar bis: 03/2021 Ch.-B: A123456

Country: Belgium

Product Code: GTIN	Sample illustration purpose
Prefix Prompts: PC: SN: EXP: Lot:	PC: 01234567890123 SN: XXX000000XXX EXP: 03/2021 Lot: A123456

Country: Bulgaria

Product Code: GTIN	Sample illustration purpose
Prefix Prompts: PC: SN: Годен до: Партида/Партиден № or Парт.№:	PC: 01234567890123 SN: XXX000000XXX Годен до: 03/2021 Парт.№: A123456

Country: Croatia

Product Code: GTIN	Sample illustration purpose	
Prefix Prompts: PC: SN: EXP or Rok valjanosti: Lot or Broj serije/Serija:	PC: 01234567890123 SN: XXX000000XXX EXP: 03/2021 Lot: A123456	

Country: Cyprus

Product Code: GTIN	Sample illustration purpose	
Prefix Prompts: PC: SN: EXP/ ΛΗΞΗ: Lot/ Παρτίδα:	PC: 01234567890123 SN: XXX000000XXX EXP: 03/2021 Lot: A123456	

Country: Czech Republic

Product Code: GTIN	Sample illustration purpose	
Prefix Prompts: PC: SN: EXP or Použitelné do: Č. Šarže:	PC: 01234567890123 SN: XXX000000XXX EXP: 03/2021 Lot: A123456	

Country: Denmark

Product Code: GTIN	Sample illustration purpose	
Prefix Prompts: PC: SN: EXP or Anvendes før Udløbsdato: Lot/Batch::	PC: 01234567890123 SN: XXX000000XXX EXP: 03/2021 Lot: A123456	

Country: Estonia

Product Code: GTIN	Sample illustration purpose	
Prefix Prompts: PC: SN: EXP or Kõlblik kuni: Lot or Partii nr:	PC: 01234567890123 SN: XXX000000XXX EXP: 03/2021 Lot: A123456	

Country: Finland

Product Code: GTIN	Sample illustration purpose	
Prefix Prompts: PC: SN: EXP or Käyt viim. Lot or Batch or Erä:	PC: 01234567890123 SN: XXX000000XXX EXP: 03/2021 Lot: A123456	

Country: France

Product Code: GTIN	Sample illustration purpose	
Prefix Prompts: PC: SN: EXP: Lot:	PC: 01234567890123 SN: XXX000000XXX EXP: 03/2021 Lot: A123456	

Country: Germany

Product Code: : NTIN for single market packs, GTIN for packs shared with other markets	**Sample illustration purpose**	
Prefix Prompts: PC: SN: Verwendbar bis: Ch.-B: NN: For multi pack markets	PC: 01234567890123 SN: XXX000000XXX Verwendbar bis: 03/2021 Ch.-B: A123456 **NN: 03389317**	

Country: Hungary

Product Code: GTIN	Sample illustration purpose	
Prefix Prompts: PC: SN: EXP or Felhasz nálható or Felh: Lot or Batch or Gy.sz.:	PC: 01234567890123 SN: XXX000000XXX EXP: 03/2021 Lot: A123456	

Country: Iceland

Product Code: GTIN	Sample illustration purpose
Prefix Prompts: PC: SN: EXP or Anvendes inden or Anv. Inden or Anvendes før Udløbsdato: Lot/Batch:	PC: 01234567890123 SN: XXX000000XXX EXP: 03/2021 Lot: A123456

Country: Ireland

Product Code: GTIN	Sample illustration purpose
Prefix Prompts: PC: SN: EXP: Lot/Batch/BN:	PC: 01234567890123 SN: XXX000000XXX EXP: 03/2021 Lot: A123456

Country: Latvia

Product Code: GTIN	Sample illustration purpose
Prefix Prompts: PC: SN: EXP or Derīgs līdz or Der.līdz: Lot or Sērija or Sēr.	PC: 01234567890123 SN: XXX000000XXX EXP: 03/2021 Lot: A123456

Country: Liechtenstein

Product Code: GTIN	Sample illustration purpose	
Prefix Prompts: PC: SN: EXP: Lot:	PC: 01234567890123 SN: XXX000000XXX EXP: 03/2021 Lot: A123456	

Country: Lithuania

Product Code: GTIN	Sample illustration purpose	
Prefix Prompts: PC: SN: EXP or Tinka iki: Lot or Serija:	PC: 01234567890123 SN: XXX000000XXX EXP: 03/2021 LOT: A123456	

Country: Luxembourg

Product Code: GTIN	Sample illustration purpose	
Prefix Prompts: PC: SN: EXP: Lot:	PC: 01234567890123 SN: XXX000000XXX EXP: 03/2021 Lot: A123456	

Country: Malta

Product Code: GTIN	Sample illustration purpose	
Prefix Prompts: PC: SN: EXP/JIS: Lot/LOTT:	PC: 01234567890123 SN: XXX000000XXX EXP: 03/2021 Lot: A123456	

Country: Netherlands

Product Code: GTIN	Sample illustration purpose	
Prefix Prompts: PC: SN: EXP/JIS: Lot or Batch or Partij or Charge:	PC: 01234567890123 SN: XXX000000XXX EXP: 03/2021 Lot: A123456	

Country: Norway

Product Code: GTIN	Sample illustration purpose	
Prefix Prompts: PC: SN: EXP: Lot:	PC: 01234567890123 SN: XXX000000XXX EXP: 03/2021 Lot: A123456	

Country: Poland

Product Code: NTIN for products registered before 2016 GTIN for all other products	Sample illustration purpose	
Prefix Prompts: PC: SN: Termin ważności or Termin ważności (EXP) or EXP: Nr serii or Nr serii (Lot) or Lot:	PC: 01234567890123 SN: XXX000000XXX EXP: 03/2021 LOT: A123456	

Country: Portugal

Product Code: GTIN	Sample illustration purpose	
Prefix Prompts: PC: SN: VAL: Lote:	PC: 01234567890123 SN: XXX000000XXX VAL: 03/2021 Lote: A123456	The 2D Data Matrix should contain a 5th element to include the national number of Portugal using the AI(714).

Country: **Romania**

Product Code: GTIN	Sample illustration purpose	
Prefix Prompts: PC: SN: EXP/Data/ expirării: Lot/Serie:	PC: 01234567890123 SN: XXX000000XXX expirării: 03/2021 Serie: A123456	

Country: **Slovakia**

Product Code: GTIN	Sample illustration purpose	
Prefix Prompts: PC: SN: EXP: Č. Šarže:	PC: 01234567890123 SN: XXX000000XXX EXP: 03/2021 Č. Šarže: A123456	

Country: **Slovenia**

Product Code: GTIN	Sample illustration purpose	
Prefix Prompts: PC: SN: EXP or Uporabno do: Lot or Številka or serije:	PC: 01234567890123 SN: XXX000000XXX EXP: 03/2021 Lot: A123456	

Country: Spain

Product Code: GTIN	Sample illustration purpose	
Prefix Prompts: PC: SN: CAD: Lote:	PC: 01234567890123 SN: XXX000000XXX CAD: 03/2021 Lote: A123456	where the GTIN14 number has to be used instead of NTIN14, the 2D Data matrix should contain additional element(s) to include national number for Spain using the AI(712).

Country: Sweden

Product Code: GTIN	Sample illustration purpose	
Prefix Prompts: PC: SN: EXP or Utg.dat.: Lot or Batch or Sats:	PC: 01234567890123 SN: XXX000000XXX EXP: 03/2021 Lot: A123456	

Country: Switzerland

Product Code: GTIN	Sample illustration purpose	
Prefix Prompts: PC: SN: EXP: Lot:	PC: 01234567890123 SN: XXX000000XXX EXP: 03/2021 Lot: A123456	

Country: United Kingdom

Product Code: GTIN	Sample illustration purpose	
Prefix Prompts: PC: SN: EXP: Lot: *UK left EU 2021	PC: 01234567890123 SN: XXX000000XXX EXP: 03/2021 Lot: A123456	

ON-BOARDING

ON-BOARDING PARTNER PORTAL

Fmd Legislation And Delegated Act

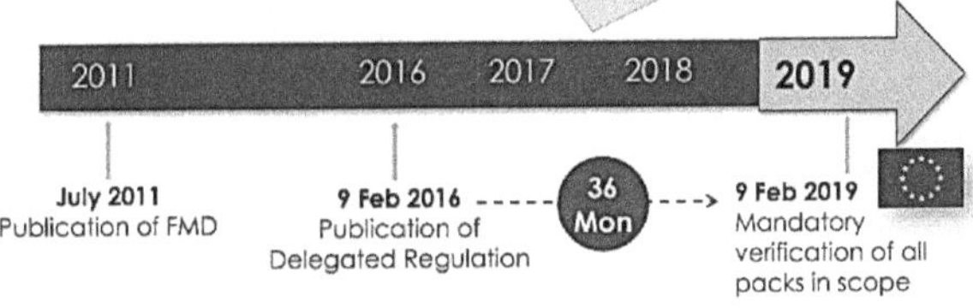

FMD: Falsified Medicines Directive

Responsibilities Of The Supply Chain Partners

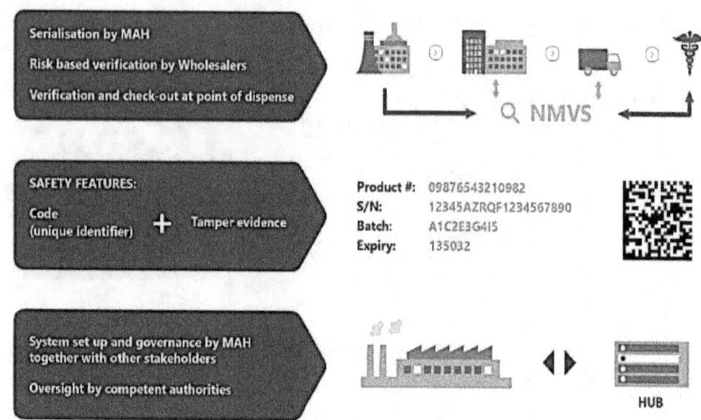

System Landscape

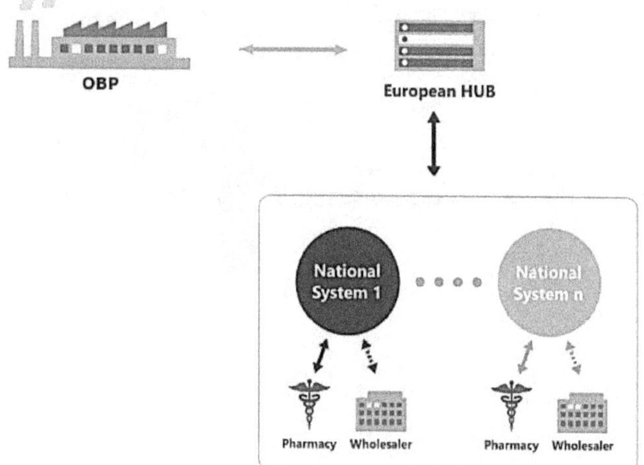

System Landscape Ii

System Landscape 2

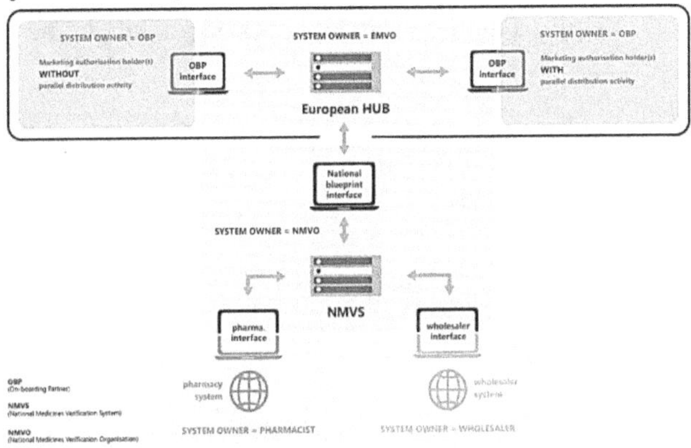

WHAT IS AN "OBP"?

- OBP means On-boarding Partner. The OBP is the contracting party of EMVO and enters into the Participation Agreement (PA) with EMVO. o The OBP represents the Marketing Authorisation Holders (MAHs) on behalf of which it will upload data on the European Hub (EU Hub).

- The OBP has therefore to be authorised to do so by its MAH/a group of MAHs.

- The OBP has to be affiliated to its MAH(s).

- The MAHs should be located in the European Economic Area (EEA).

- The OBP can only upload product data for its affiliated MAHs as long as

  - ✓ They are either original pack manufacturers or parallel distributors If the OBP would like to represent both types of MAHs, it will have to create two OBP accounts

✓ The Marketing Authorisation of the related products lies within the OBP group. Contract Manufacturing Organisations (CMOs) cannot upload their manufactured product data in the EU Hub.

Example

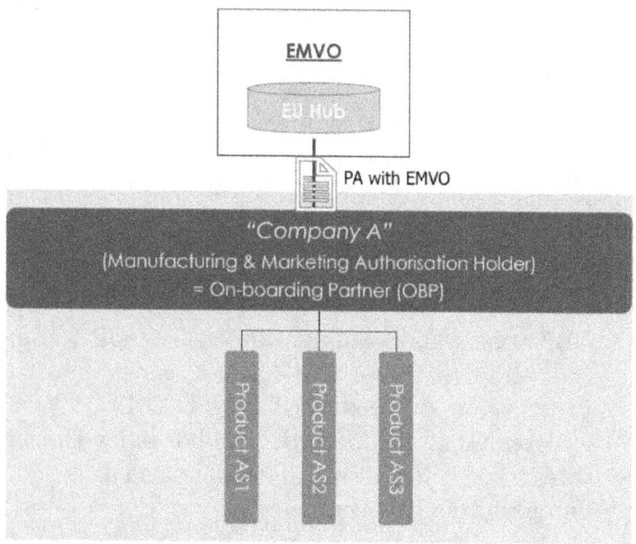

What Is An Obp Connection Provider?

- A third-party provider engaged by the OBP, who assists the OBP entirely or partially with the development, implementation, provision, use, and/or operation of the OBP interface to the EU Hub via a Gateway Connection,

- Every OBP Connection Provider has to be promoted by at least one OBP in the On-boarding Process,

- A registered OBP Connection Provider is a provider which signed the License Agreement with EMVO and a Support Contract with SolidSoft.

ON-BOARDING CONTRACT LANDSCAPE

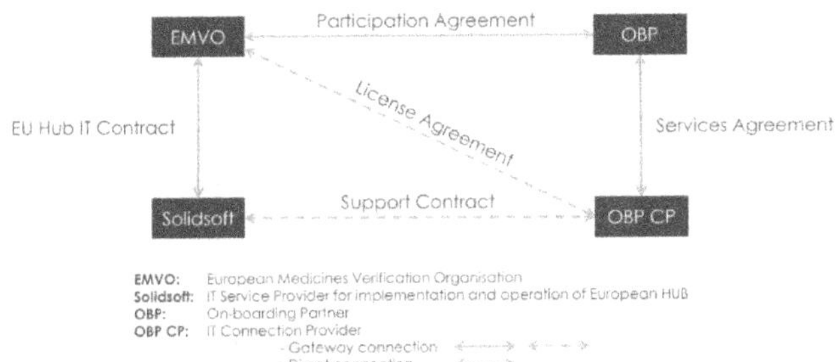

On-Boarding Process

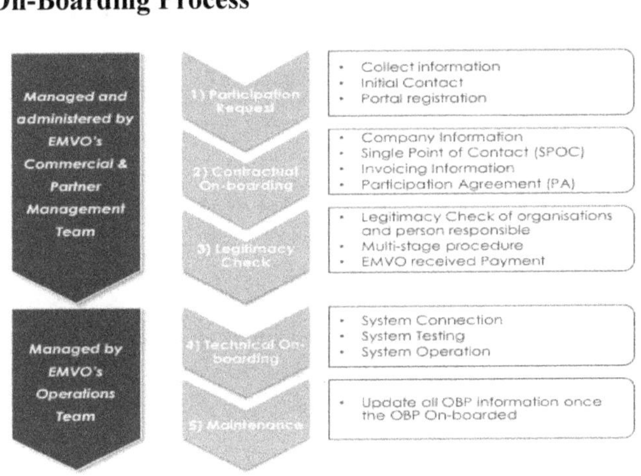

On-Boarding Partner Portal

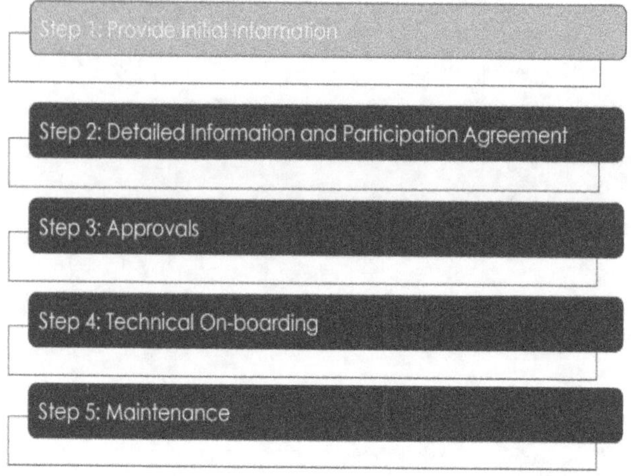

Obp Contract With Emvo
The Participation Agreement (PA)

- Contractual framework for participation in the On-boarding project, e.g. use of the EMVO Gateway, SDK*, etc
  - ✓ Interface development
  - ✓ Connect to the EU Hub

- Includes a Non-Disclosure Agreement covering the provision of Confidential Information by EMVO, e.g on
  - ✓ EU Hub
  - ✓ EMVO Gateway

- Purpose: Execution of Technical On-boarding

Emvs Master Data Guide

The EMVS (European Medicines Verification System) requires that OBP's (OnBoarding Partners) upload both product master data and product pack data.

EMVS Master Data Requirements

These consist currently of two primary data collections.

- A common 'applies to all markets' collection of data.

- A market specific collection of data.

SPOR

The long-term aim for EMVS is to have the European Hub connected to the European Medicines Agency (EMA) SPOR data repository and to use this connection to provide a source of regulatory approved data that can be utilized by EMVS to provide a higher quality of data.

The key data fields that will enable this to function, for those parties who fall under the scope of SPOR, are:

- Product Code and Coding Scheme (in EMVS)

- Data Carrier Identifier (in SPOR) which is equivalent to the Product Code in EMVS.

- ISO Country Identifier for each market of intended sale.

The highlights of the data model are as follows:

- The Common Data Section has a new 'List of ATC Codes' added. Maximum number of codes per list is ten. ATC codes can be in the 5 character format or 7 character format and they apply to all markets for the given product code. (The ATC Code cannot be updated or set directly by the OBP).

- The Product Code Status (which is not accessible by the OBP) is moved to the Market Specific Data section to support the 'Product Withdrawal' capability.

The Market Specific Data section has been upgraded to included:

- Name

- Common Name

- Pack Type

- Pharmaceutical Form

This permits the future insertion from SPOR of the localised regulatory data for each market.

Member State ISO 3166 Code

Member State ISO 3166 Code	
Austria AT	EU Master Data Guide
Belgium BE	
Bulgaria BG	
Croatia HR	
Cyprus CY	
Czech Republic CZ	
Denmark DK	
Estonia EE	
Finland FI	
France FR	
Germany DE	
Greece GR	
Hungary HU	
Iceland IS	

Ireland IE	
Italy IT	
Latvia LV	
Liechtenstein LI	
Lithuania LT	125
Luxemburg LU	
Malta MT	
Netherlands NL	
Norway NO	
Poland PL	
Portugal PT	
Romania RO	
Slovakia SK	
Slovenia SI	
Spain ES	
Sweden SE	
Switzerland CH	
United Kingdom GB	

EMVO Gateway File Input Element Name Mapping

Common EMVS Master Data Element Names	EMVO Gateway (file upload) Element Names
Product Code	CodeValue
Coding Scheme	CodeScheme
Name	Name
Common Name	CommonName
Pharmaceutical Form	FormType
Strength	Strength
Pack Type	PackType
Pack Size	PackSize
Market-Based EMVS Master Data Element Names	Market-Based EMVO Gateway (file upload) Element Names
Member state ISO Code	Id
National code	NationalCode
Article 57 code/PCID	Article57Code
	MAH
MAH ID	Id
MAH Name	Name
MAH Address (2 x Street, City, Postcode and Country Code)	Street1, Street2, City, PostCode and CountryCode
List of Wholesalers	ContractedWholesalers
Wholesalers ID	Id
Wholesalers Name	Name
Wholesalers Address(2 x Street, City, Postcode and Country Code)	Street1, Street2, City, PostCode and CountryCode

Stabilization Period (Soft lunch/implementation period)

In the proposed Stabilisation Period there should be:

- Flexible alert handling;

- Implementation of NCA reporting .

- Completion of serialization.

- Increase of EMVS stability/performance.

- Effective crisis management.

"Many countries Implemented a stabilization period to allow system and process to embed".

Alert management

Alert management: investigation efforts to focus on "potential and/or confirmed falsified medicines"

The EMVO report says: Approx. 3 % of all scans undertaken by supply chain actors lead to false alerts being generated due to various reasons, such as:

Missing data upload into the European Hub,

- Incorrect data upload,
- Incorrect scanner configuration of end-users,
- Pharmacy / hospital software systems not updated,
- Procedural reasons,
- System not used properly.

Alert Management

L5 Alert: highest level; suspected falsified medicine scanned.

- Can't dispensed to patient: firstly, fully investigated and medicine falsification has been rule out.
- L5 alert: automatically escalated to OBP and NCA required prompt action.
- Every alert means: Pack of medicine cannot be sold, potential return, customer Complaint etc.
- Handling of alert: legal obligation and now part of GMP audit scope.
- Example:
- Additional space in 2D Data Matrix Code
- The anti-tampering device is defective

Audits

- Connection with hub and On-Boarding Partner (OBP)
- Data Flow
- Generation of Serial Numbers (SNs)

- Uploading of information in the repositories system

- Application of the Anti-Tampering Device (ATD)

- Packaging Lines

- Composition, Decommissioning, status change of the Unique Identifier

- Quality of the printing of the 2D barcode

- Alert Management

Russian Track And Trace Readiness

On 1 January 2020, Russia will introduce a new, compulsory system for tracking pharmaceuticals from manufacturer to end user. This new legislation should be considered alongside wider global efforts to enhance quality control and put in place protection against fake and counterfeit medicines. Recent reports evidence the devastating impact of counterfeit medicines around the world, making the need for fully traceable pharmaceuticals more relevant than ever before.

Russian Crypto Code for Pharma Industry

Need to explain this project in 4 sections.

1. Track and Trace Serialization for Markirovka

2. The standard aggregation processes

3. The connection to MDLP (How to connect MDLP?

4. Integration with the third party softwares

What is Russia Mandate?

- From November 1, 2018, Russia's serialisation was moved under the new leadership of a new operator

CRPT. All functionalities of the systems built will remain the same so that the transition can be smooth.

- This move was to take place after Government Decree No. 791-r and No. 792-r were published. The main highlight of this decree was the introduction of crypto-codes for each pair of product code and serial number. Even though in the above-mentioned decree Medical products were not included, in August, all these doubts were put to rest with the release of the Government Decree no. 1018, which confirmed the role of CRPT as the operator of Russia Serialisation (Markirovka) from November 1, 2018

In the Russian pharmaceutical serialization regulation, unlike EU or USA , drugs are not divided to prescription and OTC. They are divided into 3 groups:

- 7VZN : The seven high-spending disease classes such as treatment of haemophilia or multiple sclerosis and patients after organ transplantation.

- ZhNVLP : Vital and essential medicines. Subject to upper price limit set by the authorities.

- All other medicines for human use.

Implementation Date for 7VZN – 01/07/2019 (*estimated)

Implementation Date for rest – 01/01/2020

Unique Identifier requirements: GS1 Unique Product code, Serial Number, 4 Digit Key (Commodity code), 44 Character signature, Batch/Expiry optional)

> *The most notable requirement in the Russian regulation is the cryptographic key which must be included in the 2D Data Matrix.*

Unit-level Packaging ("units of sale")

Barcode Symbology: Data Matrix ECC200

Barcode Contents: The "Control Identification Sign" (CIS)

- GTIN-14;

- Serial Number (13 alphanumeric characters);

- a "Crypto-code", supplied by a government service or a government supplied piece of hardware. The request for a Crypto-code must include the GTIN-14 and the Serial Number data elements because the Crypto-code are specific to those data elements;

- a 4 digit "key"

- a 44 character "signature"

	No	Application Identifier Name / AI	AI Number for GS 1	Number of Symbols	Type
Mandatory	1	GTIN	01	14	Numeric
	2	Serial Number	21	13	Alphanumeric
	3	Public Key	91	4	Alphanumeric
	4	Crypto Code / Verification Code / Private Key	92	44 or 88	Alphanumeric
Optional	6	Batch	10	Max. 20	Alphanumeric
	7	Expiry Date	17	6	Numeric
	8	Russian FEA	240	4	Alphanumeric

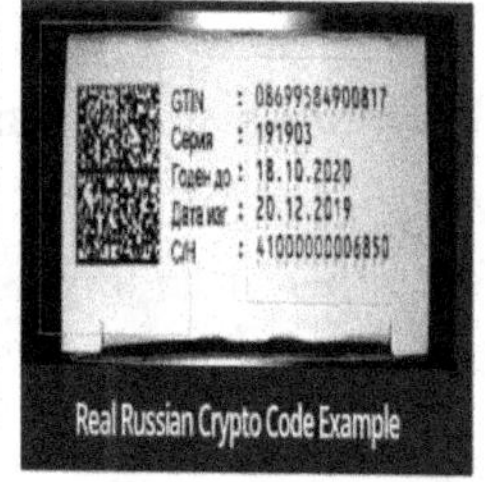

Note: Only the GTIN and serial number data elements must appear on the package in human readable form (that is, the cryptocode does not need to be printed in human readable form).

Serial Number Reuse: 5 years after issuance, or 1 year after the expiration date of the last use, whichever is later.

Connection With Mdlp

MDLP is the component of the national Chestnyy ZNAK project which has been designed for the mobility of medicines. It is specifically prepared for the pharmaceutical industries in Russia. It has a more complex infrastructure than the regulations of other countries in which the data is reported to the health authorities. To give an example, it is mandatory that each notification to the MDLP system be signed.

MDLP accommodates all the terms to trace the lifecycle of each pharmaceutical product. These terms might be listed under sub headings as follows.

1. The notification of the pharmaceutical products to the system which are produced within Russia.

2. The notification of the pharmaceutical products to the system which are imported to Russia.

3. The mobility of sales and storage

4. Extirpation and recalling.

5. Relabelling

6. Aggregation and transformation operations

7. Operation cancellations

Chestny ZNAK

Manufacturers and distributors must connect and comply with Russia's National Track and Trace Digital System, known as Chestny ZNAK but sometimes referred to as Honest SIGN and Honest BADGE.

Hallmarks include 2D Data Matrix codes, randomized serial numbers, crypto codes, unit-and batch-level trace ability, and secure reporting and records management.

No matter your role in the supply chain, it's in your interest to understand how Chestny ZNAK works and what the regulations mandate. Let's take a look.

What is Chestny ZNAK and how does it work?

Chestny ZNAK's "main objective is to guarantee the authenticity and declared quality of goods being purchased by customers.

The Center for Research in Perspective Technologies (CRPT),

Chestny ZNAK envisions a five-step track and trace process for all medicines.

First, the CRPT sends the manufacturer or importer a unique code for every product that must be affixed to the packaging. Companies must have a CRPT-authorized representative to request codes.

Second, in what's described "logistics," the digital code becomes an immutable "passport" that legitimizes the product at every node of the supply chain.

Every transfer of ownership must be recorded.

At the third juncture of the journey, when a medicine arrives at a pharmacy, hospital, clinic, or store, it's scanned and Chestny ZNAK receives a transfer confirmation. The medicine is now ready for sale.

It's important to note that Russian law requires over-the-counter (OTC) drugs to be labelled, scanned, and

132

recorded in Chestny ZNAK. This is a significant departure from regulations such as the EU Falsified Medicines Directive (FMD) and the U.S. Drug Supply Chain Security Act (DSCSA), and one reason why some in the pharma industry say the Russian regulations are too stringent.

In the last step, consumers scan the 2D codes on products using the Chestny ZNAK app for smart devices, which is in Version 4.4.0 as of March 13, 2020. It's described as "your main assistant for product quality tracking and counterfeit detection." Consumers will be the final supply chain gatekeepers.

Russian Code Structure

Russian serialization code will consist of two parts.

- Identification part: GTIN+ Serial Number
- Verification part: **Cryptographic Code**

Note: The cryptographic transformation, the data set to be coded more than doubles compared to the GS1 datamatrix used in the European Union.

Infrastructure and Crypto-System Provider

- the new operator has been the Center for Advanced Technology Development (CRPT).
- CRPT provides for allocation of crypto characters and transfer of the required data, as well as installation of Issue Recorders at the respective production sites.
- These devices will be connected to the national cloud.
- The pharma producer transmits serial numbers together with the GTIN to the cloud and in return

receives the corresponding cryptographic key for the code to be printed and verified.

- The model provides for a fee to be charged for each cryptographic key; in addition, annual maintenance costs for the Issue Recorder are under discussion.

Brazil's Track And Trace Regulations Overview

Companies selling drug product in Brazil face particularly challenging regulations, with requirements for serialization, traceability, verification, and government reporting.

A long-debated regulatory bill, PL 4069, was used as the basis for the new law, No. 13.410, which was officially signed into law and published on December 28, 2016 – setting the wheels in motion for Brazil's multi-stage implementation.

In its initial step towards serialization implementation, The SNCM was signed into law by the Brazilian Health Regulatory Agency (ANVISA) on December 28, 2016.

As per the plan, the serialization requirements were rolled out in 3 phases –

Stage 1: In September 2017, a 1-year pilot phase was initiated.

Stage 2: From September 2018 to May 2019, pilot review and the finalization of technical guidelines were done.

Stage 3: was planned for May 2019 to May 2022, including implementation of unit-level serialization.

- October 2020: Pharma stakeholders must serialize 25% of their products

- April 2021: Pharma stakeholders must serialize 50% of their product

- September 2021: Pharma stakeholders must serialize 75% of their product

- April 2022: Pharma stakeholders must serialize 100% of their product

This new law, which amends the previous regulation in Brazil, is based on extensive industry stakeholder feedback.

Brazil at a Glance

Government agency	ANVISA
Regulatory scope	Serialization; product tracking; reporting
Product scope	All pharmaceuticals, including samples; ANVISA can determine scope of medicines covered
Participants	All supply chain members
Next deadline	To be determined; in 2017, following ANVISA's completion of final rules
Serial # format	Up to 20-digit, manufacturer issued; GS1 (expected)
Reporting flow	Supply chain stakeholders to a central system accessed by ANVISA

Coding:

Unit-level Packaging ("units of sale")

Applies to: All prescription drug registration-holders (manufacturers, repackagers and importers), wholesale distributors and pharmacies.

Barcode Symbology: "DataMatrix, as specified in ISO / IEC 16022: 2006 and its updates"

Barcode Contents:

The Unique Medication Identifier (IUM), consisting of:

- Presentation GTIN (the GTIN that is drug and packaging);

- The ANVISA medication registry number for this presentation; • A unique serial number unique to this presentation;

- The expiration date of the drug

- The lot/batch number of the product.

"IUM: a series of numeric, alphanumeric or special characters, created through identification and coding standards, allowing the individualized, exclusive and unambiguous identification of each commercial packaging of the medicinal product;"

ANVISA Implementation Plan: Quick Start Guide

December 18 Update: ANVISA continues to modify its Normative Instruction and certain requirements, deadlines, and terminology may have changed since this article was originally published. Updated information will be published as soon as it becomes available.

With the 2022 ANVISA readiness deadline now less than 18 months away, ANVISA is in the final stages of finalizing its Normative Instruction and is expected to confirm its requirement that companies file their serialization implementation plans before the end of 2020.

While the Normative Instruction has not yet been formally released, it is expected that Marketing Authorization Holders (MAHs) will be required to submit a serialization implementation plan as early as December 31, 2020 via the government reporting system (SNCM) portal. In doing so, companies are signalling to ANVISA their commitment to meeting the country's track and trace requirements by February 2022.

Implementation plans must be submitted through the ANVISA portal.

Prior to the final release of the Normative Instruction, ANVISA has launched a test environment where companies can preview the web portal that they must use to submit their serialization and reporting implementation plans and register their master data:

- A valid digital certificate is required to access the portal. Individual user logins are not supported.

- Companies can track the progress of their implementation plan through a dashboard and progress chart.

- The portal will provide Portuguese, Spanish, and English language support.

- New plans can be added.

- There will be a section for companies to register serialized products that are not subject to SNCM traceability reporting.

The ANVISA web portal provides a highly structured, step-by-step process for entering company data and updating the progress of each serialization activity. Based on the final Normative **Instruction, the implementation plan must include the expected dates for the beginning and end of the following steps:**

- Process mapping

- Approval of the acquisition plan by management

- Acquisition and installation of equipment

- Packaging validation and updating of the elements of the pharmaceutical quality management system

- Integration with SNCM and logistic processes

High-level information categories include:
- **General company data**
  - ✓ Production plants
  - ✓ Total number of production lines: internal and contract manufacturing
  - ✓ Distribution centers
  - ✓ SKUs in production
  - ✓ SKUs to be serialized
  - ✓ Serialization lines for each plant

- **Implementation details for each activity, including:**
  - ✓ Start date
  - ✓ Number of days to complete
  - ✓ % completion

ANVISA has added a new metadata requirement.
ANVISA has released the technical guidelines, including a new metadata requirement and related web services and tools. This metadata links to the product's ANVISA registration number to enhance the oversight and control

capabilities of the SNCM system. Metadata can be uploaded and queried using an automated web service or by using a web interface to upload data manually using a CSV file. The required metadata includes:

- GTIN (Global Trade Item Number)
- Anatomical Therapeutic Chemical (ATC) Classification
  - ✓ ATC/WHO (World Health Organization)
  - ✓ ATC/DDD (Defined Daily Dose)
  - ✓ ATC/EphMRA (European Pharmaceutical Market Research Association)
- Portaria 344/98 Regulatory Classification / Prescription Type
- Commercialization Start Date
- Commercialization End Date (optional)
- Commercialization End Reason (optional)

ANVISA will begin automatic track and trace notifications in April 2022.

At the September 2020 SETRM conference, ANVISA noted that they will not be notifying companies of serialization or reporting issues until April 2022, when the track and trace law goes into effect. ANVISA also pointed out that there are no interdependencies between product serialization systems and the SNCM system that prevent companies from developing and registering their implementation plans and working with partners on horizontal data integration. To help companies prepare, ANVISA has created a new microsite and has published its technical guidelines for connecting and reporting to the SNCM system. In addition, they have provided a test environment to start simulating event reporting.

Serialization and Tracking/Reporting Highlights

Serialization: Brazil requires serialization at the unique item level and the transport packing container, or case, level. Aggregation is required, and each case must contain an identifier linking to the unit identifiers within that case.

Tracking and Reporting: Every member of the Brazil supply chain—manufacturers/importers, wholesale distributors, and pharmacies—must capture and store key transaction events for drug product coming into and leaving their company, as well as for certain movement and events that takes place within the company. This information must be stored for at least one year after the drug's expiration date. It is expected that all reporting will go to a centralized reporting system managed by ANVISA, but details for implementing that system are not yet determined.

Drug Serialization Requirements In China

On April 28, 2019 the Chinese National Medical Products Administration (NMPA) published two documents to clarify some of the requirements set out in the new drug traceability code.

- Encoding requirements for drug traceability code
- Guidelines for drug traceability information system construction

Coding and Serialization Requirements in China

Item level identification and traceability in China rely on three codes:

The drug traceability code is used to uniquely identify a sales package unit at each level of packaging, consisting of a list of numbers, letters, and/or symbols.

The drug identification code is a unique code used to identify a drug in regard to license holder, manufacturer, generic drug name, dosage form, formulation specifications, and package specifications.

The production identification code is a code used to identify data about the drug during the manufacturing process.

NMPA (Chinese National Medical Products Administration) advises 'issuing agencies' to define a drug traceability code generation strategy that takes into account current production needs and processes as well as future requirements (i.e. in terms of scalability, supply chain partners, etc.). The code can contain alphanumeric and special characters, should contain a check digit and be compliant with either of the 2 following:

- 20 characters with the first 7 characters being the drug identification code

- International ISO standards i.e. ISO/IEC 15459

Applies to: Marketing authorization holders, drug manufacturers, pharmaceutical operating units to establish the drug traceability systems and drug supervision and management departments of supervision and inspection. It does NOT apply to the production and operation of Chinese herbal medicines, raw materials and special packaging preparations"

Unit-level Packaging ("units of sale")

Barcode Symbology: One-dimensional barcode, two-dimensional barcode or RFID tag, etc. can be selected as the carrier of the drug traceability code according to the actual needs. Drug traceability codes shall be recognized by equipment and the human naked eyes."

Barcode Contents

The Drug Traceability Code (DTC) is a China-specific 20- character code, or any code that complies with the coding rules of relevant international standards prescribed by the International Organization for Standardization (ISO) (e.g. Standards for ISO/IEC 15459 Series)." The DTC should be associated with:

Name of the drug listing license holder

- Name of the drug manufacturer
- Generic name of the drug
- Drug approval number
- Drug standard code
- Dosage form
- Formulation specification
- Packaging specification
- Date of manufacture
- Batch
- Expiration date

And it should contain a serial number and a check digit

Unit-to-Case Aggregation Capture? : Yes

India Track And Trace System For Export Of Pharmaceuticals And Drug Consignments

Regulatory Agency: India Ministry of Commerce and Industry, Department of Commerce, Directorate General of Foreign Trade (DGFT)

DGFT: this organization has been essentially involved in the regulation and promotion of foreign trade through regulation. Keeping in line with liberalization and globalization and the overall objective of increasing of exports,

Regulation Name or System Name: Track and Trace System for Export of Pharmaceuticals and Drug Consignments

Compliance Dates: Drugs can be exported from India only if both the secondary and tertiary packaging carries the specified serialized barcode and the corresponding data is uploaded to the central portal (www.iVeda-india.in). Serializing the primary level is optional at this time.

Note: Uploading all data to the iVeda portal for production since April 1, 2022.

Barcode Symbology: Linear, or 2D Datamatrix following GS1 standards

Barcode Data Encoding: GS1 standard

Aggregation Data Capture: Yes

Authentication: Government (www.iveda-india.in for now)

- iVEDA stands for Integrated validation of exports of drugs from India and its authentication.

- Pharmaceutical exporters in India will now have to implement the Track and Trace system.

- The Central system will be *changed from DAVA to iVEDA*.

- Every company will have a profile in iVEDA portal.

- After registration and verification done Pharmexcil and user can see the dashboard.

- iVEDA developed by C-DAC will be replaced by DAVA Portal.

DAVA Portal:

- Technical glitches.

- Hampering manufactures and exporters from uploading data.

- Issues and concerns raised by pharma industries with regard to track and trace and specific reference to data upload issue in DAVA portal.

The salient features are:

- Easy Registration and Quick Verification/approvals.

- Option of aggregation/non-aggregation.

- Companies using GS1 code can continue doing so.

- Merchant Exporters can now upload the data using the necessary guidelines

- Companies can get CDAC codes in case they have not yet subscribed to get codes from GS1 or any other agencies.

- Bulk upload of XML files enabled.

The recommendations arrived after a series of consultations with the all the stakeholders led to the decision of developing a new web portal for iVEDA.

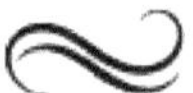

Chapter | 7

Emerging Market Regulatory Requirements

Emerging markets represent a major opportunity for pharmaceutical companies seeking revenue growth. To capture it, they need to make a rapid shift from traditional marketing and sales approaches to access-driven commercial models. Winning companies are embracing this shift as a priority in emerging markets.

SOUTH AFRICA:	
Regulation Name / Authority	Republic of South Africa - Department of Health
Serialization and Aggregation	Yes
Deadline	Jun 30, 2022
Serialization data carrier Data Elements	GS1 DataMatrix GTIN (AI 01), Batch Number (AI 10), Expiration Date (AI 17), Serial Number (AI 21),
Aggregation Data Carrier Data elements	GS1 128 Linear Barcode or GS1 Data Matrix GTIN (AI 01), Batch Number (AI 10), Expiration Date (AI 17), Serial Number (AI 21)

AUSTRALIA	
Regulation Name / Authority	Guidance on TGO 92 / Therapeutic Goods Administration (TGA)
Serialization	Yes
Deadline	Jan 01, 2023
Data carrier Data Elements	GS1 DataMatrix GTIN (AI 01), Expiration Date (AI 17), Batch/ Lot Number (AI 10) serial Number (Al 21)

BAHRAIN	
Regulation Name / Authority	System for Tracking and Tracing Medicine Provision and Supply Chain inside the Kingdom of Bahrain
Serialization and Aggregation	Yes
Deadline Serialization Deadline Aggregation	December 31, 2019 September 01, 2021
Serialization data carrier Data Elements	GS1 DataMatrix GTIN (AI 01), Serial Number (AI 21), Expiration Date (AI 17), Batch/Lot Number (AI 10)
Indonesia	
Regulation Name / Authority	National Agency of Drug and Food Control Regulation
Serialization	Yes
Deadline Serialization	JANUARY 1, 2023
Serialization data carrier Data Elements	2D Bar Code : GS1 DataMatrix GTIN - AI (01), Batch/Lot Number - AI (10), Expiration Date - AI (17), Serial Number - AI (21)

JORDAN	
Regulation Name / Authority	Guidelines of Identification and Bar coding of Medicinal Products for Human Use/JFDA
Serialization	Yes
Deadline Serialization	JAN 01, 2020
Serialization data carrier Data Elements	GS1 Data Matrix GTIN (AI 01), Serial Number (AI 21), Expiration Date (AI 17), Batch/Lot Number (AI 10)

JAPAN	
Regulation Name / Authority	Ministry for Health, Labour and Welfare (MHLW) - Japan
Serialization & Aggregation	Yes
Deadline Serialization & Aggregation	APR 01, 2021 (OR APR 01, 2023 FOR THOSE WITH SPECIAL REASONS)
Serialization data carrier Data Elements	GS1 DataBar Limited Composite Symbol CC-A, GS1 DataBar Stacked Composite Symbol CC-A, GS1 DataBar Limited or GS1 DataBar Stacked Product Code (14-digit code consisting of the JAN – Japanese Article Number) (AI 01) = uniform commodity code [UCC] Expiration Date (AI 17), Batch/Lot Number (AI 10), Serial Number (AI 21)
Aggregation Data Carrier Data Elements	GS1-128-Barcode Product Code (14-digit code consisting of the JAN – Japanese Article Number) (AI 01) Expiration Date (AI 17), Quantity (AI 30), Batch/Lot

	Number (AI 10), Serial Number (AI 21)

MALAYSIA	
Regulation Name / Authority	MoH Draft Rule
Serialization & Aggregation	Yes
Deadline Serialization & Aggregation	JAN 01, 2023
Serialization data carrier Data Elements	GS1 Data Matrix ECC200 GTIN (AI 01), Serial Number (AI 21), Expiration Date (AI 17), Batch/Lot Number (AI 10))
Aggregation data carrier Data Elements	GS1 128 SSCC (AI 00)

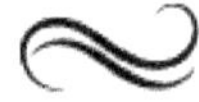

Chapter | 8

Supply Chain Digitalization

Introduction

Supply chain digitalization, or rather digital transformation, provides a path to sustainable solutions for many of the challenges in managing the pharmaceutical industry's supply chain such as *compliance, traceability, end-to-end visibility, error-reduction, quality assurance* and **process efficiencies.**

Emerging Technologies And Benefits

Whether by outsourcing or by enhancing in-house capabilities, implementing the digital transformation of the supply chains is one way for pharmaceutical companies to future–proof their operations.

It positions industry players to tackle the long-standing challenges outlined above by leveraging **Artificial Intelligence, Big Data, Predictive Analytics and Cloud computing**, all of which can lead to significant efficiencies and competitive advantages. That said, it takes efficient data integration to realise the benefits of digitalization effectively and sustainably.

End-to-end supply chain visibility, the holy grail of supply chain management, is impossible to achieve without digitalization and capturing

data from several source.

Supply chain digitalization sets in motion a virtuous cycle that will keep pharma companies future-ready and help the industry rise to the challenges of providing medicines in the 21st century. However, it is a process of many parts and getting integration right is a vital component of making digital transformation a success.

5 steps to help you improve transparency in your supply chain

basic steps you can implement to start you off on your journey.

1. Risk assessment and Setting an Outcome

2. Envision the supply chain

3. Gather information you can act on

4. Participation

5. Reporting

Those are five basic steps you can implement to improve traceability in your supply chain. Do keep in mind that supply chains are ever-changing and reacting, whether it be to changes in the economy ot new government regulations. This process to improve traceability should be ongoing and frequently reviewed. While the implementation of technology such as Blockchain can help in this matter, the final answer will entail the right balance of manpower, data, and technology which supports your desired outcome.

How to drive Successful Serialization in the Supply Chain?

The pharmaceutical industry has been able to prevent excess flooding of counterfeit and harmful products in the supply chain by ensuring compliance measures for serialization and traceability processes are followed. By implementing unique identifiers (such as unique serial numbers) for products and adhering to rules set by regulatory bodies, the industry has been able to adopt serialization for their products. This has allowed businesses to quickly identify the challenges as well as blockages in the supply chain and ensure safety for the end users.

What more can be done in the industry to improve the processes for serializing products and to build a more efficient supply chain?

1. **Strengthen data exchange networks:** Businesses can strengthen and support data exchange between various networks which can improve implementation and help them have access to accurate insights throughout the supply chain. With accurate data platforms and the right analytical tools, resources can be freed up and operations can focus on compliance and serial operations through implementing data-driven practices.

As one of the most recent trends being adopted within the pharma industry has been investing in *blockchain technology*

- **Incorporate sustainable** solutions: Sustainable digitization for packaging – this can help with anti-counterfeiting of products through serialized labels, etc.

Create sustainable strategies for increased and cost-effective ROI – this should include market changes for changing and country specific serialization regulations, supply chain interconnectivity and all future technologies in the supply chain such as the use of AI and as mentioned earlier, Blockchain.

A majority of businesses have incorporated serialization strategies in their organizations. By considering the above-mentioned processes for serializing products, the industry can look at more efficient supply chains. As the trends in technology and regulatory updates keep changing, organizations can benefit from sustainable business practices and processes of establishing data exchange networks that are interoperable. Not only does this add financial value but it also has its merits for creating a more visible, efficient and compliance driven supply chain.

A robust serialization management strategy can benefit not just the manufacturer, but the entire supply chain. With serialization of products, there's trust, responsibility, transparency and ownership between all the members (manufacturers, stakeholders and customers) in the supply chain.

How does Blockchain Technology benefit Serialization?

Blockchain Technology is a network that is decentralized and it shares real time complex information with all the participants – regulators, contract manufacturers, physicians, patients, R&D collaborators, and academic researchers, among others.

Blockchain Technology provides transparency and security to enable serialization for products. It helps with sharing vast amount of data and prevents data tampering which in return allows for regulatory auditing.

Blockchain Technology is proving to be a huge benefit in the pharmaceutical industry, especially in the following areas:

1. **Growing the Pharmaceutical Supply Chain**

2. **Transferring secure data within ecosystems**

3. **Strengthening relationships with payers**

Blockchain Technology: The Beginning of a New Era in Traceability

Imagine a traceability system without authorities, regulations, and global data providers. Give your products a unique identity and shout the data which this identity points to into space. Anyone who knows the identity can see the data you share and integrate and use it with their systems. Keep all data secure, unchangeable, transparent, and distributed. I repeat, there is no authority, no regulation, no global data providers. Isn't it like a dream?

Blockchain technology, the subject of university dissertations in the 1990s, was embodied by an academic article published by Satoshi Nakamoto in 2008. The first notable application was money that could be exchanged securely without a central bank. As you all know, it's called BitCoin. The subject of our article is a traceability system using blockchain.

Traceability in Brief

We can define traceability, in brief, as recording all the movements of a product throughout the supply chain. Today, we use traceability implementations with the pharmaceutical, food, cigarette, alcohol, and cosmetic industries.

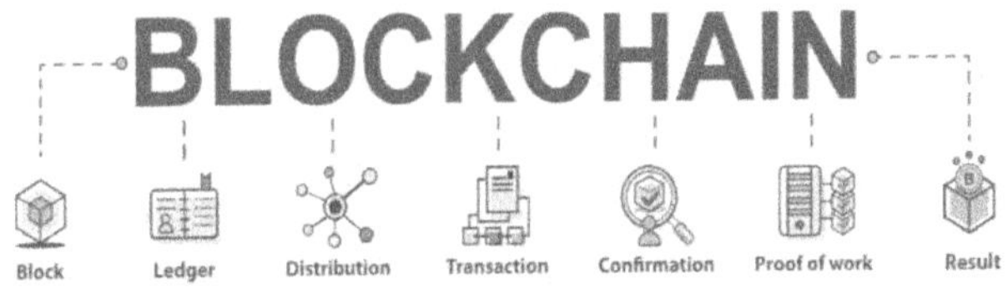

What is the Place of "BlockChain" in Traceability Implementations?

The engineering team, uncomfortable with this issue, rolled up their sleeves to create traceability systems using blockchain. They set up a big dream for a real traceability system. The dream was to record every point in the supply chain, starting with all the raw materials used in the production of a product.

Even if it seemed possible to achieve the job with conventional client-server technology, it was expensive, difficult to operate, inefficient, and boring. However, blockchain eliminated all challenges, allowing a product to be traceable throughout its lifecycle. All that needs to be done is to access the data of all the raw materials used during the production of the product from the blockchain and associate this data with a unique key that refers to the product and transfer the key to the "blockchain". No server, no authority, trust less and transparent.

traceability system established on the blockchain is much more secure than the conventional traceability system. Please note that the only way to access data in a blockchain is to have the key.

The Key to Traceability in Blockchain: Serialization

We shared which product we produced, when and where we produced it, and other information with the blockchain network (Ethereum, Ripple, Corda, etc.) to provide traceability. Well, how will our suppliers, customers, and end-users in our supply chain access this data? We called serialization the key because it's the answer to this question.

The most commonly used technologies for serialization are GS1 Data matrix and QR code. But regardless of these, we can also use techniques such as RFID, NFC, or 1D Barcode, taking into account the needs of our application. Here, it is important to present the key that will be used to access the traceability data of the product to the supply chain, taking into account user habits.

The singularization of products, especially in high-speed production lines, creates a sense of bottleneck in projects. The easiest way to overcome this feeling is to look at the development of traceability-oriented printing and image processing technologies. One of the products in the industries of ink, carbon film transfer, and laser printing that have developed with the increase of traceability requirements in the last 20 years will definitely be your solution. One of the technologies you should use to ensure that the products you serialize are traceable is image processing technology.

Blockchain In Pharma Supply Chain–Reducing Counterfeit Drugs

Experts have estimated the sale of counterfeit drugs is twice the legal pharmaceutical trade rate, which is a severe issue.

With its transparent, immutable and auditable nature, the pharma blockchain holds the potential to enhance the supply chain's

- Security
- Integrity
- Data provenance
- Functionality

Blockchain-focused companies are working on remodelling tracking and accountability in the shipping of goods.

Blockchain in Pharma Supply Chain can manage inventory as well as reduce counterfeiting and theft issues.

Here's why Pharmaceutical Supply Chain require an innovative solution:

- Visibility
- Regulatory compliances

- Cold-chain shipping

How would Blockchain-enabled pharma supply chain solution work?

Stakeholders that can be involved in the distribution of drugs are as follows:

- Manufacturers

- Logistic Service Providers

- Distributors

- Hospital/Pharmacy

- Patient

Step 1: Manufacturer manufactures the drugs and adds QR code to it

A manufacturer produces the drugs and adds the QR code to it,

The QR code contains essential information like

- timestamp

- item name

- location

- manufacturing and expiry date

The information added by the manufacturer gets stored on the blockchain, providing transparency to the supply chain to other stakeholders.

Once information is added to the blockchain, a hash ID is produced that can be used for tracking the transactions.

The drugs can be shipped to the distributors via IoT-enabled vehicles with temperature sensors to enable cold-chain shipping.

It can also be possible to exchange and store the data gathered by temperature sensors on the blockchain. In the case of an audit of temperature-sensitive drugs' storage conditions, the transparent and immutable distributed ledger can save a considerable amount of time.

The drugs transferred through IoT-enabled vehicles can also send the real-time location to the blockchain, allowing the stakeholders and government agencies to track drugs' delivery conveniently.

Step 2: Distributors send the drugs to hospitals/pharmacists

With the help of Hash ID stored on the blockchain, distributors can verify the origin of medicines after collecting them from the logistics service providers.

They can trace back the information added by manufacturers such as the date and place of manufacturing, and if it passed quality checks.

Distributors validate the received medicines and sign the transaction digitally, which is then added to the blockchain.

The signed transactions trigger the smart contracts to send drugs to the hospitals/pharmacists.

Step 3: Pharmacists receive the drugs and verify its source

Pharmacists get the drugs which can be traced back to know its origin, using the hash ID saved on the blockchain.

Suppose any illegal distributor tries to sell counterfeit drugs with fake drug ID to pharmacists or patients. In that case, the transaction is considered invalid because of the false information added about the drug.

Also, unauthorized individuals cannot carry out transactions in the drug supply chain ecosystem without a valid private key.

Therefore, pharmacists would immediately know if any anomalies are found within the transactions.

Once the pharmacist approves the received medicines, the transaction between them and the distributor is added to the blockchain, ensuring the legal deal.

Step 4: Patients buy the drugs and scan the QR code to trace back its source

Patients can ensure if the medicine they are buying is safe or not. By scanning the QR code attached to the drug's packaging via their mobile app, they can know its source and quality standards.

The hash ID linked to the QR code would fetch information from the blockchain for patients' access.

Patients can give ratings or feedback for the drugs they buy, linked to the drug's ID stored on the blockchain.

The rating added by the patient can help other individuals to decide if the specific drug is effective or not.

The drug supply chain's transaction data maintained by blockchain is consensus-driven, transparent and immutable. A blockchain-based solution can help move the governance model of the drug supply chain from regulation to surveillance net (every stakeholder can transparently survey the actions in the supply chain).

What are the benefits of blockchain's implementation in the health industry?

• End-to-end traceability of health products:

The use of a pharma blockchain based solution will enable streamlined visibility of movement and stakeholders through which drugs or medicines transit in the supply chain. The improved traceability facilitates the optimization of flows of goods and an efficient stock management system.

• Reduced losses related to counterfeiting:

A blockchain application can enable clear visualization of health product's journey from manufacturer to patients with the digitized transactions. Therefore, it would become possible to examine vulnerable points in the supply chain and reduce the chances of frauds and the costs associated with it.

• Transparency to enhance accountability:

The receiving and shipping of health products throughout the supply chain can be traced. Also, it is possible to trace the actors or stakeholders involved in the chain of shipment.

If any problem arises during the supply of drugs or medicines, blockchain can enable to identify the last stakeholder by which the product passed through.

• Efficient recall management:

Using blockchain in the pharmaceutical supply chain can allow the identification of exact locations of medicines.

The batch reminders can be sent out or carried out efficiently and quickly while maintaining increased safety of patient's health.

A private blockchain can be the compelling use case of the pharmaceutical supply chain, but the rights granted to each stakeholder can be different depending on their roles.

Real Use Cases of Blockchain Pharma Supply Chain

1. SAP Pharma Blockchain POC App

Merck is the world's oldest operating pharmaceutical company. It has developed the SAP Pharma Blockchain POC app in partnership with SAP.

SAP's existing solution wasn't blockchain-based. It was called Advanced Track and Trace for Pharmaceuticals (ATTP).

A manufacturer registers on the SAP Pharma Blockchain POC App after dispatching a bundle of pharmaceuticals. It generates:

- Item number
- Serial Number
- Batch Number
- Expiration Date

The distributor can obtain this information from the package's barcode.

Counterfeit barcodes are avoided due to the tracking feature. Also, the app allows the stakeholders to ensure that the deliveries are taking place without any oddities.

2. **Novartis Blockchain**

Novartis is currently in the process of launching an IoT and blockchain-based solution for tracking temperature and identifying counterfeit medicines. The project leaders are Marco Cuomo and Daniel Fritz. It plans to launch it by the end of 2020.

Novartis is also the lead industry in forming a 29-member blockchain consortium for the European Union and the European pharmaceutical industry. Earlier known as the Innovative Medicine Initiative (IMI), it is now known as Pharmaledger. It was formed in January 2020.

3. **TraceRx**

Developed by LeewayHertz Technologies, TraceRx is a distributed ledger platform that enables traceability of shipment of drugs and solves thefts, recalls and transparency in the medicine shipments.

Our team of blockchain development experts provided a blockchain solution that helped our client empower the entire drug supply chain with enhanced tracking and traceability.

How Artificial Intelligence Is Improving The Pharma Supply Chain

The AI transformation goes much deeper than smarter search functions. It holds the potential to address some of the biggest challenges in pharmaceutical cold chain management. Here are some examples:

Analytical decision-making: a drug order and weather data along a delivery route, for example — AI-based systems can provide complete visibility with predictive data throughout the cold chain.

Supply chain management (SCM): for better transparency around costs, logistics, warehousing and inventory. Assuring drug efficacy, patient identity and chain of custody integrated with supply chain agility is where the true value of AI lies for the drug industry.

Inventory management: pharmaceutical companies must stock many more therapeutics but in much lower quantities. AI-based inventory management can determine which product is most likely to be needed (and how often), track exactly when it's delivered to a patient, and provide delivery time and delays or incidents that might trigger replacement shipment within hours.

Chapter | 9

Definitions And Abbreviations

1. **GS1 DataMatrix 2-D Barcode:** The GS1 DataMatrix barcode is a graphic representation of digital data in a two-dimensional format with high information-decoding capacity.

2. **Global Trade Item Number (GTIN):** The GS1 Global Trade Item Number (GTIN) is an identification key that uniquely identifies products worldwide. It can be encoded in various types of data carriers, including GS1 DataMatrix.

3. **Global Location Number (GLN):** The global location number (GLN) is a globally unique GS1 identification number that can identify any location in the supply chain that needs to be uniquely identified.

4. **Serial Number (SN):** The serialization number (SN) is used to identify each product unit of product identified by GTIN. The SN used for a product cannot be used again for the same product. The SN can be up to 20 alphanumeric characters in length.

5. **Application Identifier (AI) :** The field of two or more digits at the beginning of an element string that uniquely defines its format and meaning.

6. **Attribute :** An element string that provides additional information about an entity identified with a GS1 identification key, such as batch number associated with a Global Trade Item Number (GTIN).

7. **Batch Number:** The batch or lot number associates an item with information the manufacturer considers relevant for traceability of the trade item. The data may refer to the trade item itself or to items contained in it.

8. **Data Carriers:** Different kinds of media that can hold GS1 Identification keys and application identifiers.

9. **Expiry Date:** An expiration date or expiry date is a date after which a product should no longer be used, either by law or by exceeding the anticipated shelf life for perishable goods.

10. **Primary Packaging:** The first level of packaging for the product marked with an automatic identification and data carrier (AIDC) either on the packaging or on a label affixed to the packaging.

11. **Secondary Packaging:** A level of packaging marked with an automatic identification and data carrier (AIDC) that may contain one or more primary packages or a group of primary packages containing a single item

12. **Scanner:** An electronic device to read barcode and convert them into electrical signals understandable by a computer device

13. **3PL Third-Party Logistics** : A contracted company that provides distribution services of finished goods on behalf of another company. A 3PL never takes ownership of the product although the product is in its possession.

14. **3PP:** Third Party Printer. An organization that's contracted to print serial numbers onto packaging containers.

15. **ADR:** Authorized Distributor of Record. A wholesale distributor that a manufacturer designates or authorizes to distribute its products.

16. **Aggregation:** The process of recording the serial number of a container along with the serial numbers of its contents; often referred to as a parent/child relationship, or a serialized container to content relationship.

17. **Alphanumeric:** Character set made up of digits and letters of the alphabet

18. **Asynchronous Transactions:** Transactions that do not have to be completed before another transaction can be processed.

19. **Authenticate:** The practice of checking a unique identifer against a set of captured serialized data to determine its authenticity.

20. **B2B:** Business-to-Business. Interactions that support the transfer of standardized interchange files up to an enterprise's EDI system. B2B interactions are not

integrated with manufacturing, warehouse, or other backend business systems.

21. **Case:** A container of product cartons which may or may not be bundled.

22. **Check Digit:** Redundancy check used for error detection of identification numbers. Used in NDCs, DEA numbers, GTIN-14 identifiers, and SSCCs, for example.

23. **Commission:** Process of associating a unique identifier to a particular object (product, shipment, asset, or container).

24. **CSV:** Comma Separated Values. A common data exchange format stored in a tabular format. CSV files can be opened in spreadsheet programs.

25. **Decommission:** The process of removing a unique identifier from a product or container so it is no longer tracked. Unlike the business process known as destroying, the item may still physically exist after decommissioning even though it no longer carries serialized identification.

26. **Destroy:** In instances where a product or container no longer exists, the process of removing a unique identifier from that item so it is no longer tracked.

27. **Disaggregation:** Removing products or containers from their associated parent container. The serial numbers of the contained items are no longer associated as children of the parent container.

28. **Disposition:** The state of a serial number, such as commissioned or decommissioned.

29. **DQSA:** The Drug Quality and Security Act. U.S. Federal legislation passed in November 2013.

30. **DSCSA:** The Drug Supply Chain Security Act, which is Title II of DQSA. DSCSA mandates a full supply chain traceability system from pharmaceutical manufacturer to pharmacy dispenser for prescription drugs being distributed in the United States

31. **ECC:** Error Correction Coding. A code applied to transferred data for error control. Provides redundancy and allows the receiver to recover the original data.

32. **EDI:** Electronic Data Interchange. The electronic transfer of data between computer systems in a standardized message format.

33. **EPC:** Electronic Product Code. A unique number that identifies a specific item in the supply chain. Also known as a serial number.

34. **EPCglobal:** The organization developing standards for the Electronic Product Code (EPC), and for RFID systems to store and manage EPCs. EPC Global is sponsored by GS1.

35. **EPCIS:** Electronic Product Code Information Services. A GS1 EPCglobal standard designed to enable EPC-related data-sharing within and across enterprises. This data-sharing is aimed at enabling participants in the EPCglobal Network to obtain a common view of the disposition of EPC-bearing objects within a business context.

36. **European Hub:** A cloud-based gateway for EU compliance reporting. Provides interoperability

between different national systems in the EU, and managing product status (such as decommissioning and recalls) and exceptions throughout the life cycle of a product. The hub doesn't store serialization data like a repository – instead it acts as a single point of entry.

37. **FMD:** The Falsified Medicines Directive. A pan-European directive, also referred to as EU FMD, intended to protect patients from counterfeit medicines in the legal distribution chain. The European Medicines Verification System (EMVS) was developed to implement the FMD.

38. **GS1 Company Prefix:** A globally unique identifier for a company, assigned and administered by GS1 Global. The GS1 Company Prefix is 4 to 12 digits, and is a component of GLN, GTIN, and SSCC identifiers.

39. **GCP:** Global Company Prefix. A globally unique code that is used to represent a location in identifiers. See also GS1 Company Prefix.

40. **HDA (formerly HDMA):** Healthcare Distribution Alliance (formerly the Healthcare Distribution Management Association). The national association in the U.S. representing primary, full-service healthcare distributors. HDA member companies deliver more than nine million prescription medicines and healthcare products to more than 165,000 settings fraudulent transaction, or (d) appears otherwise unfit for distribution such that the product would be reasonably likely to result in serious adverse health consequences or death to humans.

41. **HRI:** Human Readable Interpretation. Characters, such as letters and numbers, which can be read by people and are encoded in data carriers. HRI is a one-to-one illustration of the encoded data.

42. **Illegitimate Product:** Defined by the FDA as a product for which credible evidence shows that it (a) is counterfeit, diverted, or stolen, (b) is intentionally adulterated such that the product would result in serious adverse health consequences or death to humans, (c) is the subject of a components and documentation needed for continued operation are installed and in place.

43. **Internal Material Number:** A number assigned to a product for internal use and not for identifying the product externally.

44. **Interoperability:** The ability of technology systems and software to communicate, exchange data and/or information, and make use of the information that's been exchanged.

45. **L1 – L5:** The 5 levels of serialization and information management: L5 – Network-level serialization system, L4 – Enterprise serialization system, L3 – Site-level serialization, L2 – Packaging line software, L1 – Device.

46. **MAH:** Marketing Authorization Holder. The license holder (brand owner) of a pharmaceutical product.

47. **Master Data :** Data representing a company's details, global identifiers, products, and trading partners. Particular types of data are required for serialization and global compliance reporting.:

48. **National System:** An information system set up and governed by national stakeholders to ensure a medicine's authenticity by verifying its safety features, to prevent falsified products from entering the supply chain.

49. **NDC:** National Drug Code. A unique 10-digit product identifier for human drugs in the U.S. Represents the labeler or vendor, the product, and the package size. Some government agencies have adopted 11-digit NDCs by padding the identifier with leading zeros.

50. **Parallel Importer:** An organization that buys a product on the open market with the intention to repackage or relabel, and then distributes it outside the network that's set up by the manufacturer or that manufacturer's authorized distributor

51. **Pedigree:** A certified record that contains information about each distribution of a prescription drug. It records the sale of an item by a manufacturer, any acquisitions and sales by wholesalers or repackagers, and final sale to a pharmacy or other entity administering or dispensing the drug. The process generally begins with the serialization of a product, and then continues through the supply chain as the product is received by each trading partner.

52. **Recall:** The removal of a drug product from the market. In the U.S., recalls fall under three classifications: Class I is for those products that can probably lead to adverse health effects or death; Class II is for drugs that can cause temporary or reversible

health effects; and, Class III relates to instances where the drug is not likely to cause adverse health effects.

53. **RFID:** Radio-Frequency Identification. The use of an object, typically referred to as an RFID tag, applied to or incorporated into a product, animal, or person, for the purpose of identification and tracking using radio waves.

54. **Safety Feature:** Elements, such as anti-tampering devices and barcodes carrying product and pack data, that are incorporated into a medicine product's packaging and identification to facilitate verification. Under FMD, for instance, safety features contain a) a unique identifier encoded in a 2D barcode, and b) anti-tampering technologies.

55. **Serial Number:** Typically a portion or component of a Unique Identifier (UID) which provides uniqueness. Also known as a serial reference.

56. **sFTP:** Secure File Transfer Protocol. A network protocol that provides file access, transfer, and management over a secure channel.

57. **sGTIN:** Serialized Global Trading Item Number. The combination of a Global Trade Identification Number and a serial number which uniquely identify an item.

58. **Site Server:** A computer system located in a specific locale responsible for a location-specific function. In traceability systems, site servers usually refer to local servers which allocate serial numbers to packaging control systems and/or manage serial number information before it is transmitted to an enterprise traceability event repository.

59. **SOAP:** Simple Object Access Protocol. A messaging protocol for exchanging structured (XML) information in the implementation of web services.

60. **SSCC:** Serial Shipping Container Code. A GS1 standard used in logistic encoding and communications. The SSCC ensures that logistic units are identified with a number that is unique worldwide

61. **T3:** Under DSCSA, the combination of Transaction Information (TI), Transaction History (TH), and the Transaction Statement (TS) for a drug product as it moves through the drug supply chain.

62. **TPM:** Third-Party Manufacturer. A company contracted to manufacture drug product for a brand owner. Also referred to as a contract manufacturer, Contract Manufacturing Organization (CMO), or Third-Party Packager (3PP).

63. **Track and Trace:** The process of tracking drugs through the supply chain using serialization data. Track and trace systems begin with serialization but generally include additional components such as product tracing or tracking, verification, and/or reporting.

64. **UID:** Unique Identifier. A string of numbers and characters that is unique within a given system. Examples include GS1 GTIN and GS1 SSCC identifiers.

65. **XSD:** XML Schema Definition. Describes the structure of an XML document.

References:

1. Georgiana Andreea Pascu, Gabriel Hancu, Aura Rusu; Pharmaceutical Serialization, a Global Effort to Combat Counterfeit Medicines; Seria Medica 2020;66(4):132-139

2. Bulletin of the World Health Organization, Volume 88, number 4, April 2010, http://www.who.int/bulletin/volumes/88/4/10020410/en/index.htm

3. History of track and trace & future of serialisation - EPM Magazine

4. Stefan Hockenberger; Track & Trace with SAP Solutions Book; pg.12-43

5. Track and Trace Obstacles, Solutions and Benefits | Pharmaceutical Track & Trace System (drugtrackandtrace.com)

6. Pharma Serialization - The Most Comprehensive Description | VISIOTT

7. Serialisation in the Pharmaceutical Industry – What You Need to Know – SL Controls

8. Serialization in the Pharmaceutical: Improving Track and Trace (xcelpros.com)

9. Serialization: What It Means for Pharmaceutical Manufacturing (aniglobalsource.com)

10. Pharma serialisation reconciliation: a blind spot in your finished product's manufacturing compliance? (europeanpharmaceuticalreview.com)

11. What would we mean if we said rfxcel was an L1-L5 solution provider?

12. What is Aggregation in Serialisation and Why Is It Important? – SL Controls

13. The GS1 System of Standards (gs1hk.org)

14. Implementation Guideline (gs1.org)

15. Anatomy of a GTIN – RxTrace

16. Fundamentals of the Pharmaceutical Supply Chain (pharmanewsintel.com)

17. How can Serialization Management enhance your Supply Chain? - Cosmotrace

18. How to drive Successful Serialization in the Supply Chain? - Cosmotrace

19. 5 steps to help you improve transparency in your supply chain - Cosmotrace

20. How does Blockchain Technology benefit Serialization? - Cosmotrace

21. Supply Chain Analytics | Supply Chain Visibility | NeuroTags

22. White+Paper+-+DSCSA_MDM_Center+for+Supply+Chain+Studies_FINAL.pdf (squarespace.com)

23. Master Data 101 What it is and How it Impacts Serialization (tracelink-quality-portal.com)

24. master-data-serialization-ebook.pdf (tracelink.com)

25. Master Data Exchange for Serialization and Track and Trace | TraceLink

26. Serial Number Manager | TraceLink

27. Serial Number Exchange | TraceLink

28. Serialized Operations Manager | TraceLink

29. Serialization Profile - SAP Help Portal

30. Serialization Pharma: Requirements for pharmaceuticals (wipotec-ocs.com)

31. Serialisation Requirements in the Pharmaceutical Industry (pharmout.net)

32. Drug Supply Chain Security Act (DSCSA) | FDA

33. United States Department of Health and Human Services - Wikipedia

34. What We Do | FDA

35. Drug Quality and Security Act - Wikipedia

36. DSCSA : Serialization Requirements and Deadlines (adents.com)

37. PowerPoint Presentation (fdli.org)

38. PowerPoint Presentation (nacds.org)

39. PowerPoint Presentation (gs1.org)

40. DSCSA Solution Including Serialization & Aggregation (visiott.com)

41. EU FMD – Anti-Counterfeiting, Identification, and Brand Protection Solutions (pharmasecure.com)

42. Falsified medicines: overview | European Medicines Agency (europa.eu)

43. European-Pack-Coding-Guideline-V4_0.pdf (emvo-medicines.eu)

44. EMVO_0086_OBP On-boarding Presentation (emvo-medicines.eu)

45. EMVO_0122_EMVS Master Data Guide (emvo-medicines.eu)

46. [Industry Update] Global Serialization: Russian Track and Trace Readiness | Pharma Logistics (pharmalogisticsiq.com)

47. Russia Serialization – Anti-Counterfeiting, Identification, and Brand Protection Solutions (pharmasecure.com)

48. Serialization Regulation Update: Russia Adopts the "Crypto-code" Law | WIPOTEC-OCS (wipotec-ocs.com)

49. An Overview of Russia's Pharma Serialization Regulations and its National Track and Trace Digital System, Chestny ZNAK | World Pharma Today

50. Russian Crypto Code for Pharmaceutical Industry - VISIOTT Technologie

51. Microsoft Word - Systech-Russia-RegUpdate_08-2020.docx (hubspot.net)

52. Brazil ANVISA Update: New Proposal for Serialization Implementation – Anti-Counterfeiting, Identification, and Brand Protection Solutions (pharmasecure.com)

53. Brazil Pharmaceutical Serialization Regulations | TraceLink (tracelink-quality-portal.com)

54. Your ANVISA Implementation Plan: Quick Start Guide | TraceLink

55. Timeline for Brazil Serialization Requirements (rfxcel.com)

56. Microsoft Word - Systech Brazil RegUpdate_08-2020.docx (systechone.com)

57. Drug Serialization Requirements in China: New Guidance Documents (adents.com)

58. Microsoft Word - Systech-China-RegUpdate_08-2020.docx (systechone.com)

59. Directorate General of Foreign Trade | Ministry of Commerce and Industry | Government of India (dgft.gov.in)

60. Microsoft Word - Systech-India-RegUpdate_08-2020.docx (hubspot.net)

61. IVEDA (iveda-india.in)

62. Serialisation: South Africa will join the fight against counterfeiting | WIPOTEC-OCS (wipotec-ocs.com)

63. tqs-infographic.pdf (serialization-pharma.com)

64. Making pharma industry future-proof through supply chain digitalization (tss.se)

65. 5 steps to help you improve transparency in your supply chain - Cosmotrace

66. How to drive Successful Serialization in the Supply Chain? - Cosmotrace

67. How does Blockchain Technology benefit Serialization? - Cosmotrace

68. Blockchain Technology : The Beginning of a New Era in Traceability (visiott.com)

69. Blockchain in Pharma Supply Chain - Reducing Counterfeit Drugs (leewayhertz.com)

70. How Artificial Intelligence Is Improving the Pharma Supply Chain (modality-solutions.com)

71. PPR_Guideline_Medicines Barcoding and Serialization Guidelines 2019_V1.2_20190520.pdf (nhra.bh)

72. 144-must-know-terms-to-decipher-serialization.pdf (tracelink.com)